LENRY LO

HIIT workout 5 minutes a day!

Transform your body with this powerful workout. Achieve impressive results and sculpt your physique using the incredible power of HIIT training.

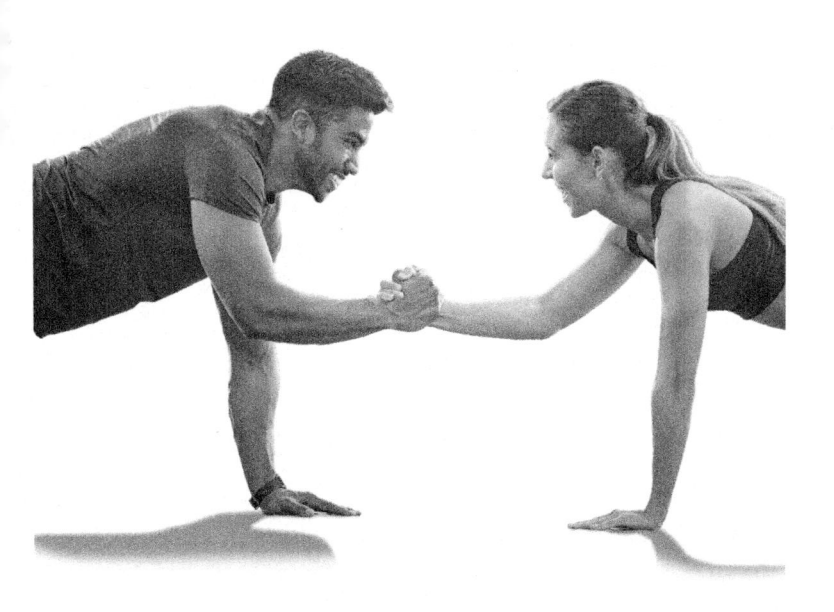

starting level: FOR ALL

Copyright © 2023 Lenry Lombardo

All rights reserved.

No part of this book may be reproduced or transmitted in any form or by any means, whether electronic or mechanical, including photocopying, recording, or any information storage and retrieval system, without the written permission of the author, except for brief quotations used in critical articles and reviews.

INDICE

Introduction _____ page 4

Chapter 1: My Personal Journey
to Body Toning with HIIT Training _____ page 6

Chapter 2: Preparing for HIIT Training _____ page 13

Chapter 3: 5-Minute HIIT Workout Sessions __ page 14

- Session 1: Fat Burning with
  High-Intensity Exercises _____ page 18

- Session 2: Building and Toning Muscles
  with Targeted Exercises _____ page 37

- Session 3: Comprehensive Circuits for
  Total Body Engagement _____ page 55

- Session 4: Interval Training for
  Full Body Muscle Work _____ page 72

- Session 5: Advanced HIIT Workout
  to Challenge Your Limits _____ page 90

Chapter 4: Tracking Your Progress _____ pag 111

Chapter 5: Nutrition and Supplementati _____ page 113

Chapter 6: Recovery and Overall Well-being _ page 116

Chapter 7: Sustaining Long-Term Results ____ page 119

Conclusion _____ page 121

Author information _____ page 123

INTRODUCTION

Hello everyone!

I am excited to share with you my approach to HIIT training, a revolutionary method to tone your body in just 5 minutes a day. But before we dive into the world of high-intensity fitness, let me explain why HIIT stands out from other fitness programs.

When it comes to achieving our fitness goals, we are often told that we must spend hours and hours in the gym, dedicating ourselves to long and repetitive workouts. However, HIIT training is different. It is based on a short yet intense approach, alternating periods of maximum effort with brief periods of active recovery.

The true magic of HIIT training lies in its effect on our metabolism. During a HIIT workout session, our bodies are pushed to the maximum levels of effort, stimulating the cardiovascular system and putting our metabolism into fat-burning mode. This means that we will continue to burn calories even after finishing the workout, thanks to the increase in post-exercise energy consumption.

But that's not all: HIIT training not only helps us burn

fat but also develops and tones our muscles. The high-intensity movements engage multiple muscle groups simultaneously, providing a full-body workout. Additionally, the high intensity of HIIT training stimulates the production of anabolic hormones, which promote muscle growth and definition.

The beauty of HIIT training is that it only requires a few minutes a day. It's perfect for anyone with a busy lifestyle and limited time for exercise. In just 5 minutes, you can achieve the same benefits as a longer workout, if not even better.

So, if you are ready to take a step forward in your fitness journey, join me as we explore HIIT training together to burn fat, build muscle, and achieve a toned and fit body.

Get ready to discover a completely new way of exercising that will save you time and bring you extraordinary results. I can't wait to share with you the workout sessions and secrets I have learned along my personal journey.

Get ready to transform your body in just 5 minutes a day!

CHAPTER 1: MY PERSONAL JOURNEY TO BODY TONING WITH HIIT TRAINING

Hello everyone! I'm excited to share with you my experience with HIIT training, a revolutionary method for toning the body in just 5 minutes a day. Before delving into the world of high-intensity fitness, let me explain why HIIT stands out among other workout programs.

In my quest for an effective and time-efficient training method, I stumbled upon HIIT. I was tired of spending countless hours at the gym with minimal results. I yearned for something different, something that could rapidly and effectively transform my body.

Enter HIIT training. It became a pivotal moment in my fitness journey. I discovered that dedicating just 5 minutes a day to HIIT could yield astonishing results. This approach allowed me to burn fat and build muscles more efficiently than I had ever imagined.

Throughout my personal HIIT journey, I witnessed a significant transformation in my physique. I began to notice increased muscle definition and a reduction in body fat. However, it wasn't solely about the physical changes. I felt more energized, resilient, and self-assured. HIIT training pushed me to new and exhilarating heights, with each session becoming an opportunity to exceed my previous limits.

Learning to manage the intensity and tailor exercises to my abilities was crucial, enabling me to make the most of these short yet intense workouts. It's important to acknowledge that my HIIT journey came with challenges. There was a learning curve, and I discovered the significance of listening to my body and allowing ample time for recovery. Balancing training with proper nutrition and adopting active recovery strategies played a key role in maximizing my results.

Today, thanks to HIIT training, I've achieved a toned and fit body without devoting hours to workouts. I take immense pride in my accomplishments and aspire to share my journey with others, believing that HIIT training can profoundly impact those seeking a swift and effective path to fitness.

Through this book, my aim is to guide you on your body toning journey with HIIT training. Sharing my knowledge, experiences, and advice, I hope to inspire and motivate you to embrace the extraordinary benefits of training for just 5 minutes a day. Are you ready to join me on this transformative journey? Get prepared to reshape your body quickly and effectively with HIIT training!

Chapter 1: Understanding HIIT - High-Intensity Interval Training

Hi everyone! I'm thrilled to introduce you to the world of High-Intensity Interval Training, commonly known as HIIT. This workout method revolves around short bursts of intense effort followed by active or complete recovery periods. It's the intensity that makes HIIT so special and effective for body toning.

During a HIIT workout, we challenge our bodies with exercises that push us to our limits, testing our endurance and strength. These exercises can include sprints, jumps, squats, push-ups, and more, tailored to our preferences and goals.

The secret to HIIT lies in its intensity. During the high-intensity intervals, we give it our all, pushing ourselves to the max. This elevated effort stimulates our metabolism, promoting fat burning even after we finish the workout, an effect known as the "afterburn." The active or complete recovery periods give our bodies a brief rest before tackling another round of intense effort. This work and recovery cycle repeats throughout the workout, which can last anywhere from a few minutes to around twenty minutes, depending on our preferences and fitness level.

HIIT training offers an array of benefits. Apart from effectively burning fat, it improves cardiovascular endurance, muscle strength, and metabolic balance. Furthermore, since it's a short-duration workout, HIIT easily fits into our daily routines, making it easier to stay consistent and motivated in achieving our body toning goals.

Personally, HIIT training has brought me visible and tangible results in terms of muscle definition and body fat loss. It's been both a physical and mental challenge, pushing me beyond my limits and helping me reach new milestones.

Throughout the rest of this book, we'll dive deeper into the principles and techniques of HIIT training, providing practical advice on creating effective workout sessions tailored to our individual needs. I'm excited to share the secrets and strategies I've learned during my personal HIIT journey.

Are you ready to explore everything there is to know about HIIT training and transform your body in just 5 minutes a day? Well then, let's get started!

2: Key Principles of HIIT Training for Optimal Results

HIIT training is centered around key principles that are crucial for achieving the best possible outcomes. Understanding and applying these principles can significantly enhance the benefits of HIIT for body toning.

Intensity: Intensity lies at the core of HIIT training. During the periods of maximum effort, it is essential to give it your all, pushing yourself to the limit. This stimulates your metabolism and promotes fat loss. The goal is to go all-out during each work interval.

Interval Duration: The duration of effort and recovery intervals varies based on personal preferences and fitness levels. Typically, effort intervals are shorter, ranging from 20 to 60 seconds, while recovery intervals can be slightly longer, between 30 and 90 seconds. Striking the right balance between work and recovery is vital to optimize the effectiveness of the training.

Exercise Variation: Varying the exercises during an HIIT workout is vital. This prevents your body from adapting and targets different muscle groups, providing a comprehensive and balanced workout. Experimenting with a variety of exercises, such as sprints, jumps, squats, and push-ups, helps engage your entire body and achieve the best possible results.

Gradual Progression: HIIT training can be highly intense, so it's crucial to progress gradually. Start with intensity and duration levels that match your fitness level and gradually increase the challenge over time. This allows your body to adapt and improve without risking injuries or exhaustion.

Recovery and Rest: Recovery and rest are essential components of HIIT training. After an intense workout, it's crucial to allow your body the time it needs to recover and regenerate. Ensure you allocate enough rest days between HIIT training sessions to prevent fatigue and promote muscle repair.

By following these key principles of HIIT training, I have experienced remarkable results in my body toning journey. Embracing the right intensity, interval duration, exercise variation, gradual progression, and proper recovery will enable you to maximize the benefits of HIIT and efficiently achieve your fitness goals. Get ready to challenge yourself and surpass your limits as you discover the transformative potential of HIIT training!

Chapter 3: Structure of a HIIT Workout: Combining Intensity and Recovery

The structure of a HIIT workout is essential to maximize its benefits. It revolves around a dynamic balance between intensity and recovery, pushing our bodies to achieve new levels of performance.

During a HIIT workout, we alternate between short bursts of maximum effort and active or complete recovery periods. The effort intervals demand our utmost commitment and intensity, pushing our physical limits. This activates our metabolism and promotes fat burning while improving endurance and strength.

On the other hand, the recovery periods allow us to briefly recuperate before facing the next round of intense effort. Active recovery involves low-intensity exercises or light movements to maintain blood flow and elevate heart rate. Complete recovery, instead, involves total rest, allowing the body to fully recover before the next effort interval. The duration and intensity of these intervals can vary based on personal preferences and fitness levels. You can start with shorter intervals, like 20 seconds of effort followed by 40 seconds of recovery, and gradually increase as your endurance and strength improve.

The HIIT workout structure offers numerous advantages. Apart from effective fat burning, it improves cardiorespiratory capacity, increases muscle strength, and promotes muscle growth. Additionally, HIIT training is highly flexible, fitting into our daily routines, enabling us to achieve significant results in a short time.

Personally, I find the combination of intensity and recovery in HIIT training extremely rewarding. Each session challenges me to surpass my previous limits and give it my all.

Throughout the rest of the book, we'll delve into various HIIT workout structures, providing practical tips for creating effective and stimulating sessions. It's important to experiment and find what works best for you, considering your fitness levels and preferences.

Get ready to strategically combine intensity and recovery as we explore different HIIT training methods. You'll be amazed by the results you can achieve in just 5 minutes a day, pushing your body towards new milestones of toning and fitness.

Are you up for this challenge? Let's get started!

CHAPTER 2: PREPARING FOR HIIT TRAINING

If there's one thing I've learned during my HIIT training journey, it's the vital importance of proper preparation before the workout. One of the key pillars of this preparation is a well-executed warm-up. Warming up before HIIT training is absolutely essential to readying my body for the intense physical activity that follows.

The warm-up routine starts with a few minutes of light cardio, such as jogging in place or jumping rope. This helps to elevate body temperature, improve blood circulation, and prime my cardiovascular system for the upcoming exertion. After the cardio phase, I shift my focus to specific warm-up exercises that target the muscle groups involved in the workout. Dynamic stretching exercises like lunges, joint rotations, and movements involving major joints are incorporated. Additionally, I incorporate mobility exercises to enhance flexibility and range of motion.

Proper warm-up yields numerous benefits. Firstly, it increases muscle and connective tissue elasticity, significantly reducing the risk of muscle and ligament injuries during the workout. Moreover, it enhances coordination and movement precision, allowing me to perform exercises more efficiently and effectively.

In addition to warm-up, I also take other precautions to ensure a safe and productive HIIT training session. Ensuring proper posture and technique during each exercise is paramount. Correct posture not only prevents injuries but also optimizes the execution of each movement. Additionally, I listen closely to my body during the workout. If I experience any pain or discomfort during an exercise, I immediately stop and assess the situation. It's crucial to respect the body's signals and avoid pushing beyond my limits.

Lastly, maintaining proper hydration throughout the entire workout is crucial. Drinking water at regular intervals helps maintain fluid balance and prevents dehydration, which could negatively impact performance and overall well-being.

Properly preparing for HIIT training and taking the necessary precautions for safety are fundamental to enjoying an effective and risk-free workout. Whether you're a beginner or an experienced athlete, following these guidelines will help you maximize results and get the most out of your HIIT training.

Here are three examples of warm-up routines you can perform before starting your HIIT workout:

1 - CARDIOVASCULAR WARM-UP:

Skipping: Run in place, lifting your knees high, for about 1-2 minutes.

Jumping Jacks: Do a series of jumping jacks for 1-2 minutes.

Jump Rope: Jump rope for 1-2 minutes.

2 - JOINT MOBILITY WARM-UP:

Joint Rotations: Perform circular movements with your shoulders, arms, legs, and ankles to improve joint mobility.

Trunk Twists: Stand with your feet shoulder-width apart, rotate your torso to the right and left to loosen the spine.

Leg Flexions and Extensions: Lie on your back, flex and extend your legs to relax the leg muscles.

3 - DYNAMIC WARM-UP:

Alternating Lunges: Take forward steps with one foot at a time, bending the knees and keeping the torso upright. Alternate sides for 1-2 minutes.

Arm Circles: Extend your arms laterally and make circular movements forward and backward to loosen the shoulders and arms.

Heel Touches: Run in place while trying to touch your heels with your glutes, maintaining a moderate pace for 1-2 minutes.

Make sure to dedicate at least 5-10 minutes to warming up to raise your body's temperature, improve blood circulation, and prepare your muscles for high-intensity training.

CHAPTER 3: 5-MINUTE HIIT WORKOUT SESSIONS

5-minute HIIT workout sessions are an effective way to achieve significant results in a short amount of time. These brief bursts of intensity can make a difference in body toning and overall fitness improvement. During these workout sessions, I focus on high-intensity exercises that engage the entire body. The goal is to push myself to the maximum during each interval, alternating moments of intense effort with short periods of active recovery.

The 5-minute HIIT workout sessions are perfect for days when I have limited time or to add an extra touch of intensity to my regular training routine. Despite their short duration, these sessions are extremely effective in burning fat, boosting metabolism, and building muscle.

The key to getting the most out of these workout sessions is to give my all during each interval. I

commit to 100% effort and push beyond my limits, knowing that every minute counts. My aim is to work hard throughout the allotted time, striving to surpass my previous results each time.

The 5-minute HIIT workout sessions can include a variety of exercises, such as squats, lunges, push-ups, mountain climbers, burpees, and many others. The important thing is to maintain a high pace and perform the exercises with proper technique. Despite their brevity, these workout sessions can be challenging and demanding. However, the sense of accomplishment and the feeling of having given my best are incredibly rewarding.

So, when time is limited but I want significant results, I rely on 5-minute HIIT workout sessions. I focus on intensity, push beyond my limits, and appreciate the benefits that this type of training can offer. Now that we have explored the 5-minute HIIT workout sessions, let's continue on our journey of toning and muscle development.

Session 1: Fat Burning with High-Intensity Exercises

Session 1 is dedicated to burning fat through high-intensity exercises. This session is perfect for boosting metabolism and accelerating body fat loss. Here's how I structure my session:

Description: In this session, I train with a series of full-body exercises, such as burpees, jumping jacks, jump squats, and mountain climbers. These exercises are dynamic, engaging multiple muscle groups simultaneously, and increasing heart rate.

Timing: Each exercise is performed for 40/50 seconds, followed by 10/20 seconds of active recovery, such as jogging in place or light walking. The complete session lasts 4/5 minutes. (Each exercise duration may vary based on the specific exercise type.)

Difficulty: Session 1 can be challenging, especially if you are new to high-intensity training. However, you can adjust the intensity based on your abilities. Start with a moderate pace and gradually increase intensity as you build endurance.

Exercise Order: You can follow the suggested exercise order below or modify it according to your preferences.

SHEET 1 - GOAL: BURNING FAT WITH HIGH-INTENSITY WORKOUT.

50" exercise - 10" active rest = 4 minutes

1 - Burpees with 2
possible alternatives:
High Knees and Jumping Lunges

2 - Jumping Jacks

3 - Jump Squat

4 - Mountain Climbers

EXERCISES AND DESCRIPTIONS:

1 - Burpees: Start in a standing position. Perform a push-up, then jump into a squat position, and finally, leap up with arms raised overhead. Repeat the movement throughout the exercise duration.

→

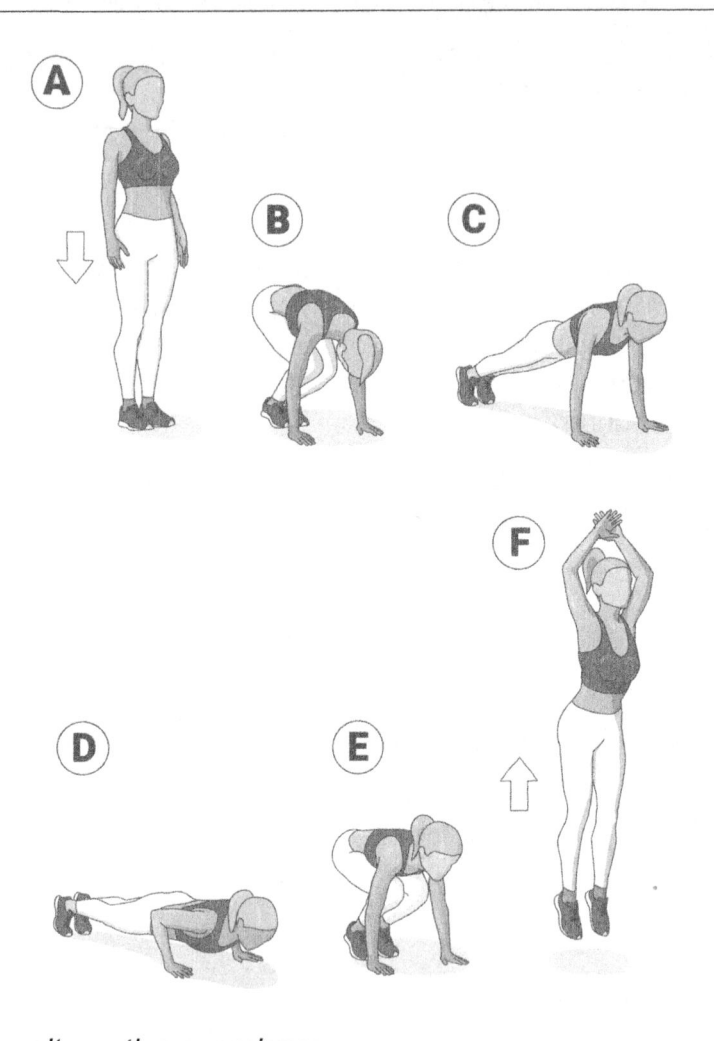

Two alternative exercises:

High Knees (Alternative): Begin in a standing position with arms relaxed at the sides. Take a step forward, raising one knee high towards the chest while simultaneously lifting the opposite arm upward. Quickly alternate legs, maintaining a fast pace and aiming to lift the knees as high as possible. This exercise engages the abs, legs, and improves cardiovascular endurance.

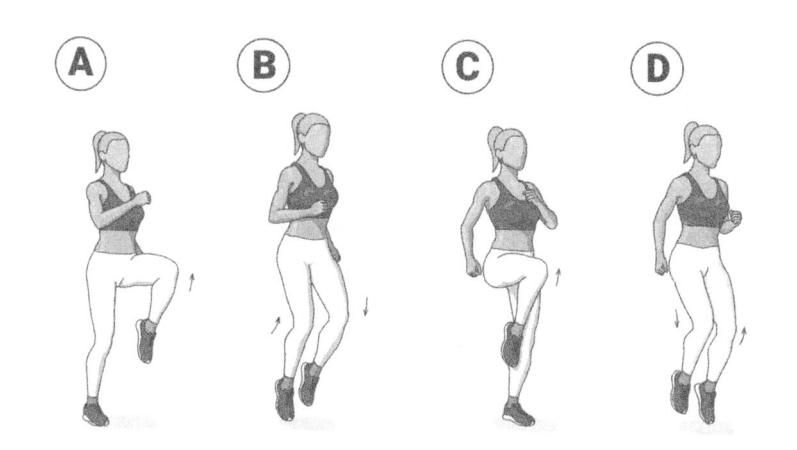

Jumping Lunges (Alternative): Start in a standing position with one foot forward and the other back in a lunge position. Jump, switching the positions of the legs, so that the foot that was forward is now back, and vice versa. Keep switching legs with a fast and controlled jump.

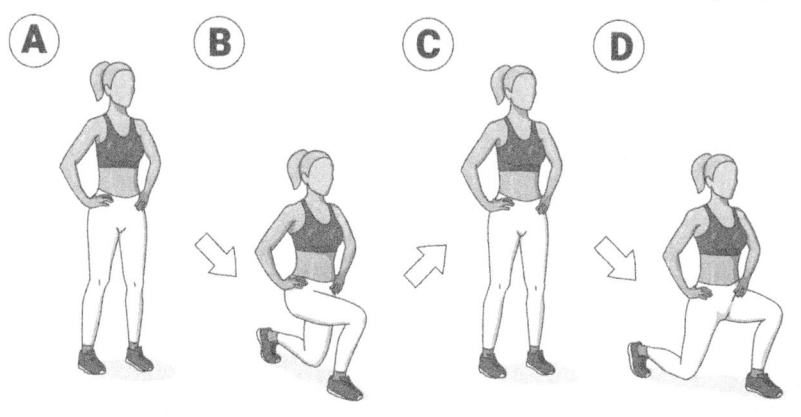

2 - Jumping Jacks: Begin in a standing position with legs together and arms down at the sides. Then jump, spreading the legs laterally and raising the arms overhead. Return to the starting position and repeat the movement for the entire exercise duration.

→

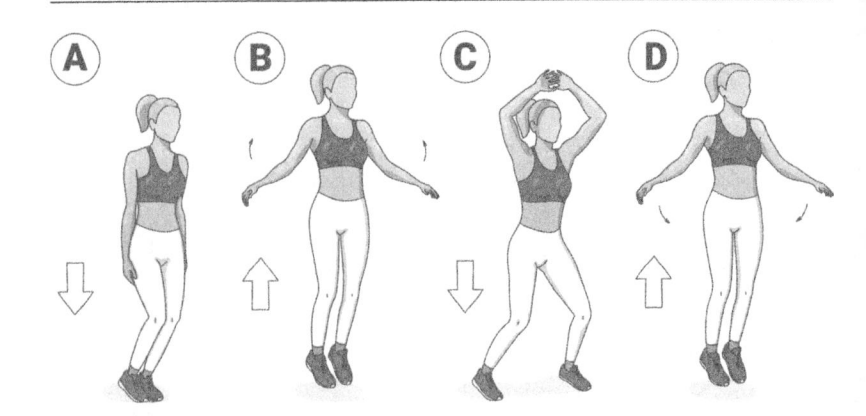

3 - Jump Squat: Start in a standing position, then jump up and land in a squat position. Jump again to return to the standing position and repeat the movement throughout the exercise duration.

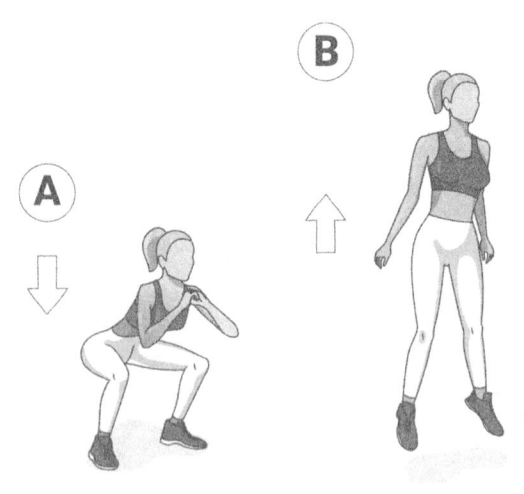

4 - Mountain Climbers: Start in a plank position, then quickly and controlledly bring the knees alternately towards the chest. Keep alternating legs throughout the exercise duration.

(A) (B)

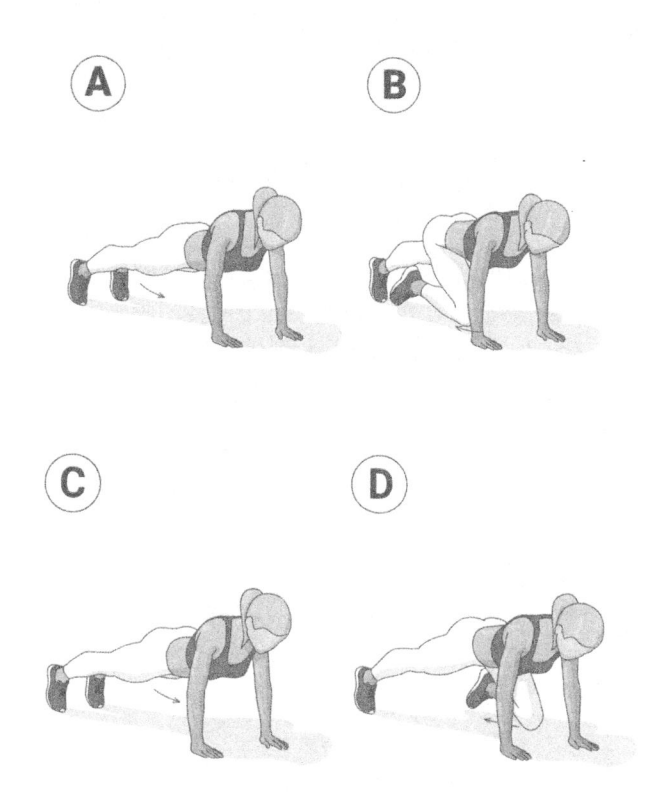

(C) (D)

Remember to adjust the intensity of the exercises according to your physical abilities and perform a proper warm-up before starting the workout.

SHEET 2 - GOAL: ACHIEVE FAT BURNING THROUGH A HIGH-INTENSITY WORKOUT.

50" exercise - 10" active rest = 5 minutes

1 - Jumping Jacks

2 - Lunges with Knee Drive

3 - Plank Jacks with Push-up

4 - Squats

5 - Knee to Elbow

EXERCISE DESCRIPTIONS:

1 - Jumping Jacks: Begin in a standing position with legs together and arms down at the sides. Then jump, spreading the legs laterally and raising the arms overhead. Return to the starting position and repeat the movement for the entire exercise duration.

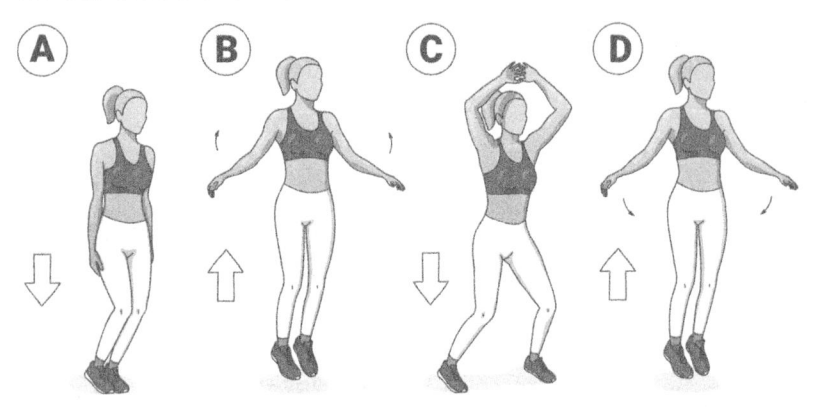

2 - Lunges with Knee Drive: Begin by standing with your feet shoulder-width apart. Take a step forward with your right foot, bending both knees to lower yourself towards the floor. Push your body upward, focusing on the front leg, and bring your left knee toward your chest during the upward motion. Alternate sides by stepping forward with your left foot and bringing your right knee toward your chest during the upward motion.

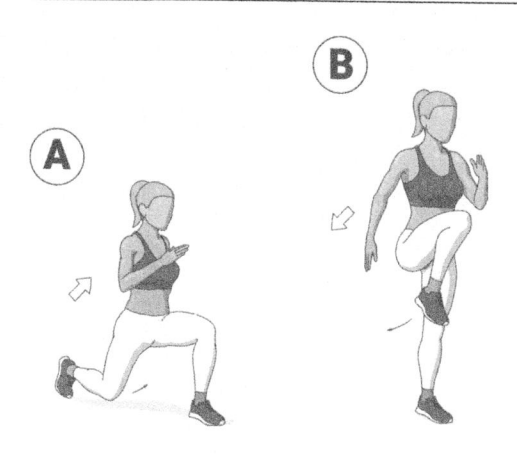

3 - Plank Jacks with Push-up: Start in a plank position with your arms extended and your body in a straight line. Jump your feet apart, then perform a push-up. Repeat this movement smoothly for the entire exercise duration.

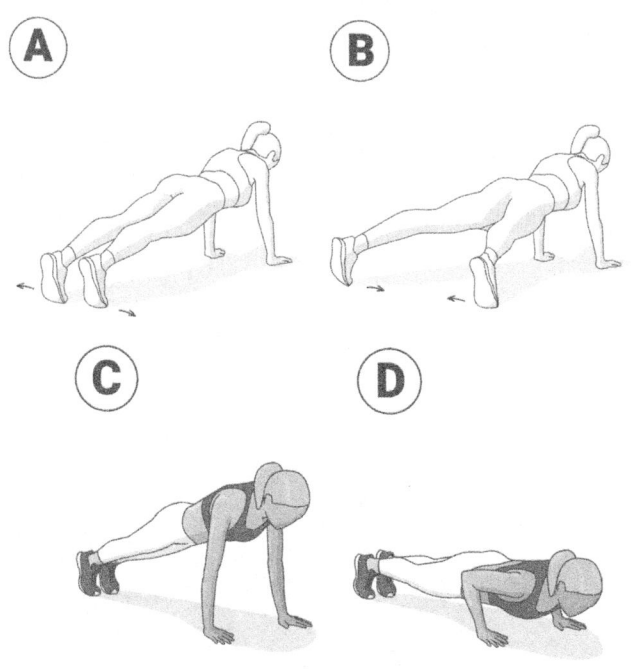

4 - Squats: Begin by standing upright, then bend your knees and lower your body as if you were sitting on an imaginary chair. Ensure your back remains straight, and your weight is distributed evenly on your heels. Repeat this movement for the entire exercise duration.

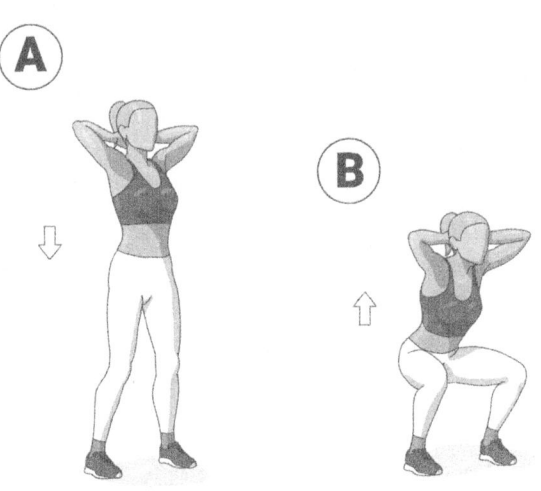

5 - Knee to Elbow: Assume a plank position while bringing your knee close to your elbow. This exercise engages your oblique abdominal muscles and core, promoting fat burning.

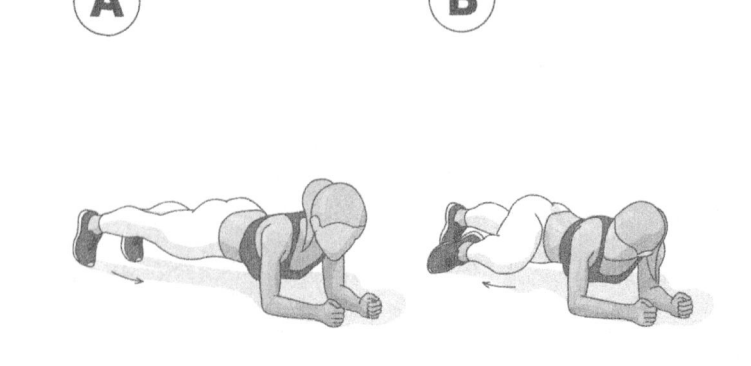

© D

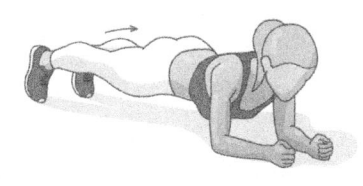

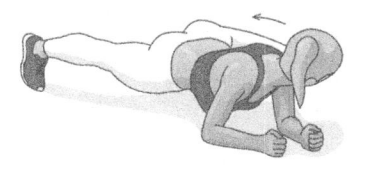

Remember to adjust the exercise intensity to match your physical abilities and always perform a proper warm-up before starting your workout.

SHEET 3 - OBJECTIVE: ACHIEVE FAT BURNING THROUGH A HIGH-INTENSITY WORKOUT.

50" exercise - 10" active rest = 5 minutes

1 - Crunches (Abdominals)

2 - Push-up with Mountain Climber

3 - Plank Walk

4 - Swimmer

5 - Plank Shoulder Taps

EXERCISE DESCRIPTIONS:

1 - Crunches (Abdominals): You can choose the type of abdominal exercise you prefer, such as crunches, sit-ups, or bicycle crunches. Focus on engaging your abdominal muscles and maintain proper form.

→

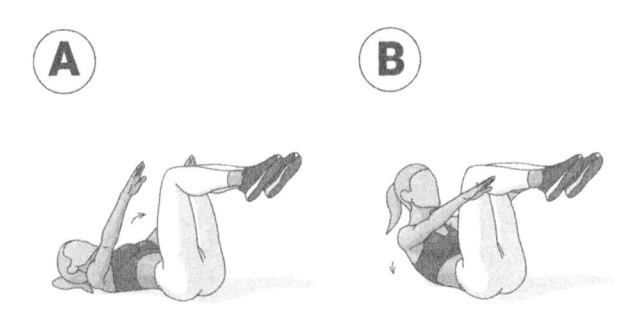

2 - Push-up with Mountain Climber: Begin with a push-up on the ground, then, as you return to the plank position, alternately bring your right knee and left knee towards your chest at a brisk pace. Continue this leg alternation throughout the exercise.

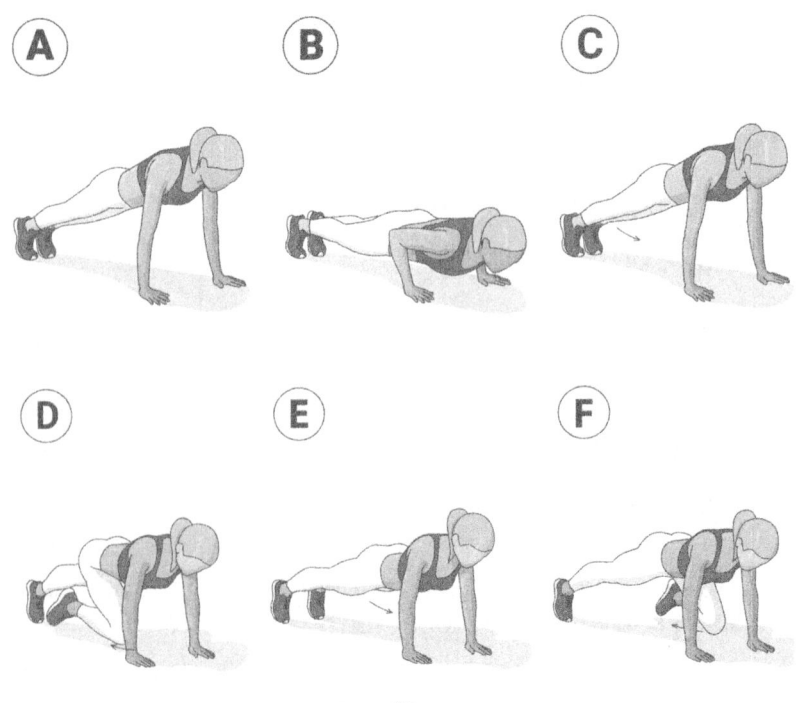

3 - Plank Walk: Engage in a walking movement while in the plank position, involving your core, arms, and legs. This exercise enhances stability and calorie burning.

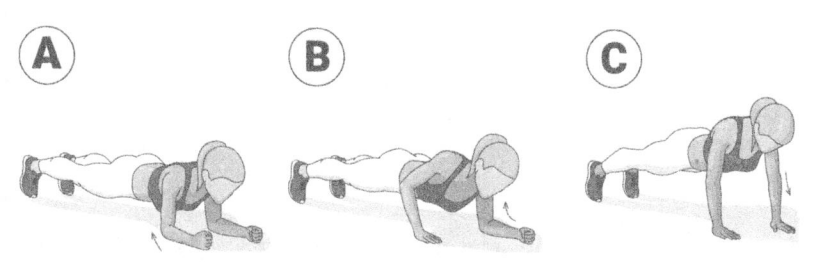

4 - Swimmer: This exercise mimics the motions of swimming and engages your core, arms, and legs. It promotes fat burning and increases muscle endurance.

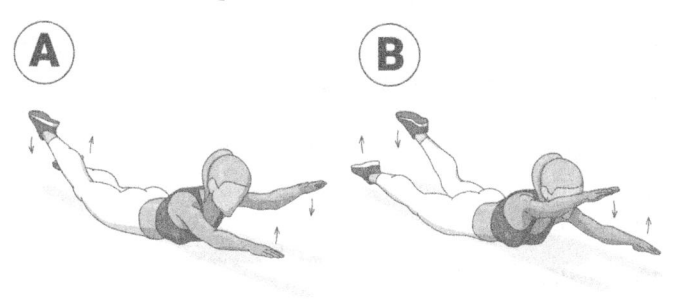

5 - Plank Shoulder Taps: Assume a plank position and alternate tapping your shoulders. This targets your abs, oblique abdominals, and activates the shoulder stabilizers.

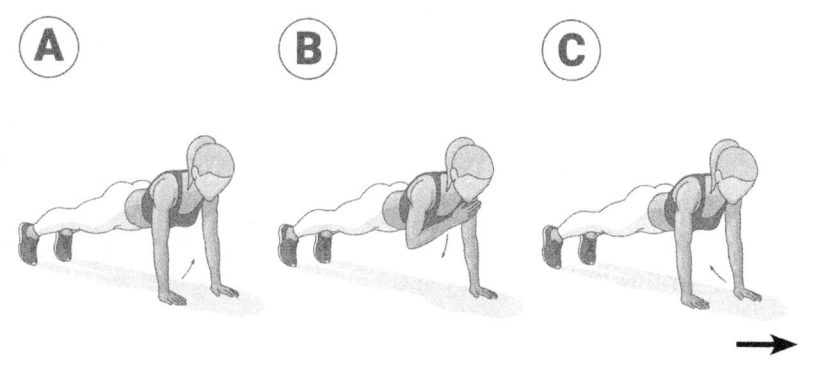

(D)

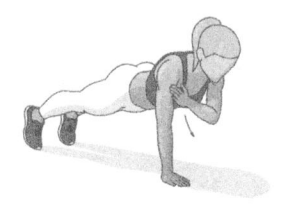

Remember to adjust the exercise intensity to match your physical capabilities and to perform a proper warm-up before beginning your workout.

SHEET 4 - OBJECTIVE: ACHIEVE FAT BURNING THROUGH A HIGH-INTENSITY WORKOUT.

50" exercise - 10" active rest = 5 minutes

1 - Jumping Jacks

2 - Mountain Climbers

3 - Traditional Lunges

4 - Flutter Kicks

5 - Plank

EXERCISE DESCRIPTIONS:

1 - Jumping Jacks: Begin in a standing position with legs together and arms down at the sides. Then jump, spreading the legs laterally and raising the arms overhead. Return to the starting position and repeat the movement for the entire exercise duration.

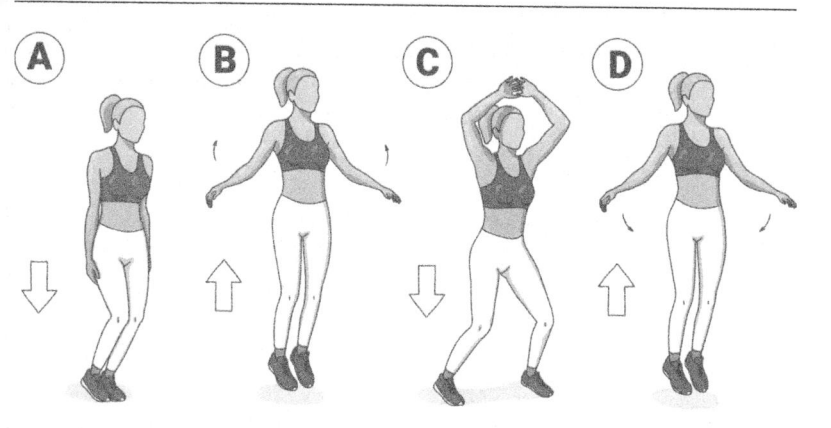

2 - Mountain Climbers: Start in a plank position, then quickly and controlledly bring the knees alternately towards the chest. Keep alternating legs throughout the exercise duration.

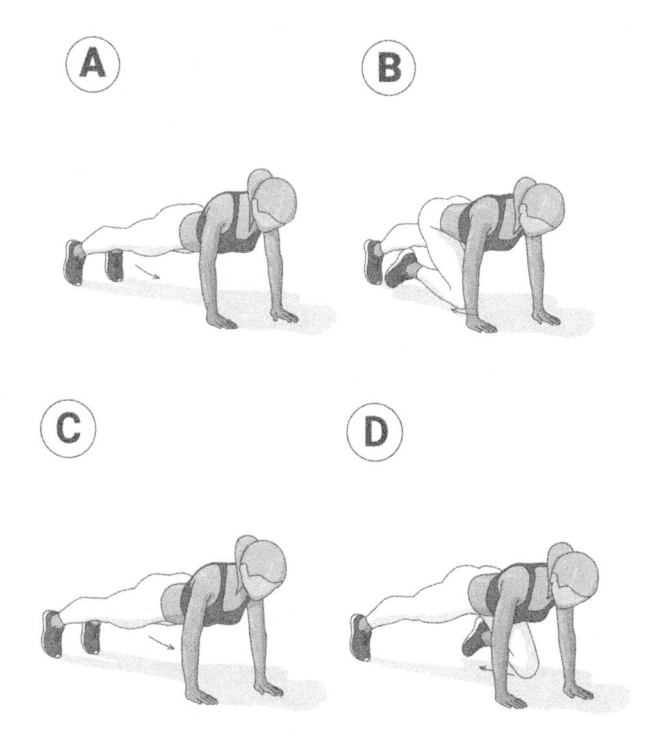

3 - Traditional Lunges: Perform classic lunges, engaging the leg and glute muscles while increasing your heart rate and burning calories.

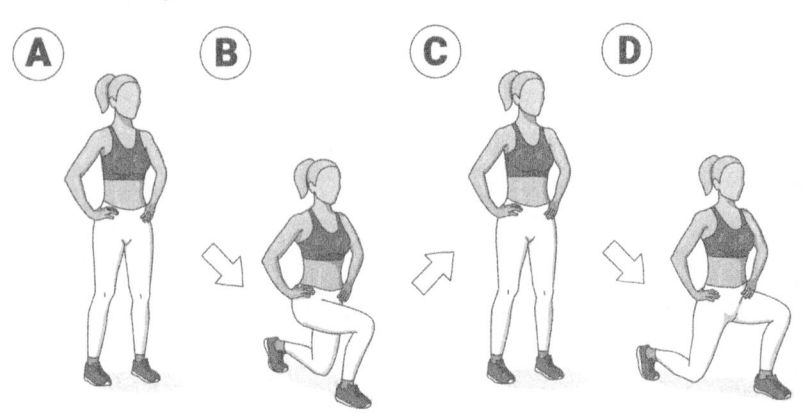

4 - Flutter Kicks: Lie on your back and lift your legs in a fluttering motion. This targets your lower abdominal muscles, leg muscles, and helps burn calories.

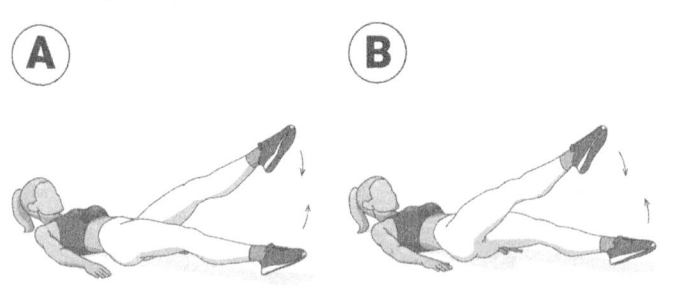

5 - Plank: Assume a static plank position, engaging your abdominal, leg, and arm muscles while stabilizing your core. You can choose between the two options provided.

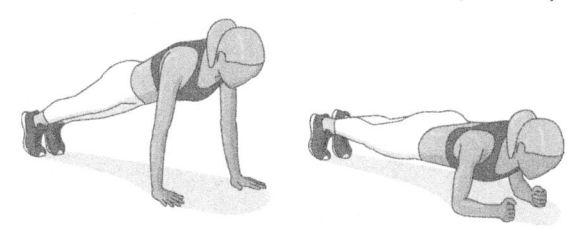

Remember to adjust the exercise intensity to match your physical abilities and perform a proper warm-up before starting your workout.

SHEET 5 - OBJECTIVE: ACHIEVE FAT BURNING WITH A HIGH-INTENSITY WORKOUT.

50" exercise - 10" active rest = 5 minutes

1 - Jump Squats

2 - Plank Jack with Push-up

3 - Mountain Climbers

4 - Plank

5 - Plank Walk

EXERCISES AND DESCRIPTIONS:

1 - Jump Squats: Perform a squat followed by a high jump. This activates leg, glute, and abdominal muscles, boosting endurance and calorie burn.

→

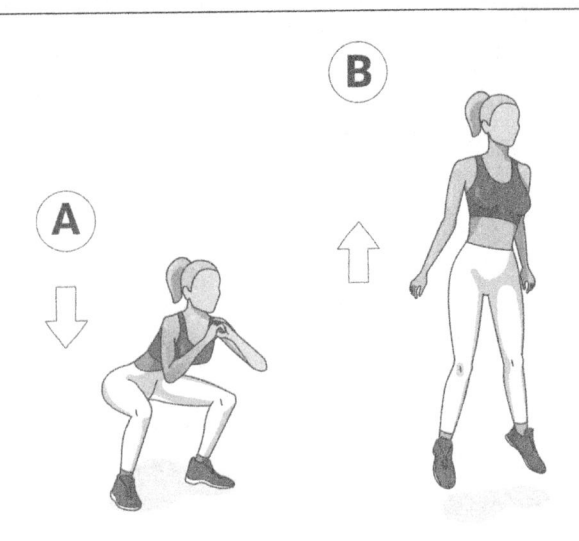

2 - Plank Jacks with Push-up: Start in a plank position with your arms extended and your body in a straight line. Jump your feet apart, then perform a push-up. Repeat this movement smoothly for the entire exercise duration.

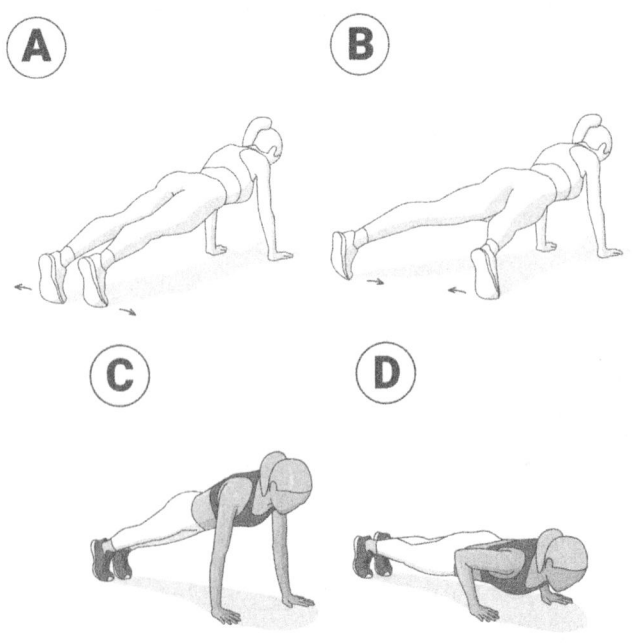

3 - Mountain Climbers: Start in a plank position, then quickly and controlledly bring the knees alternately towards the chest. Keep alternating legs throughout the exercise duration.

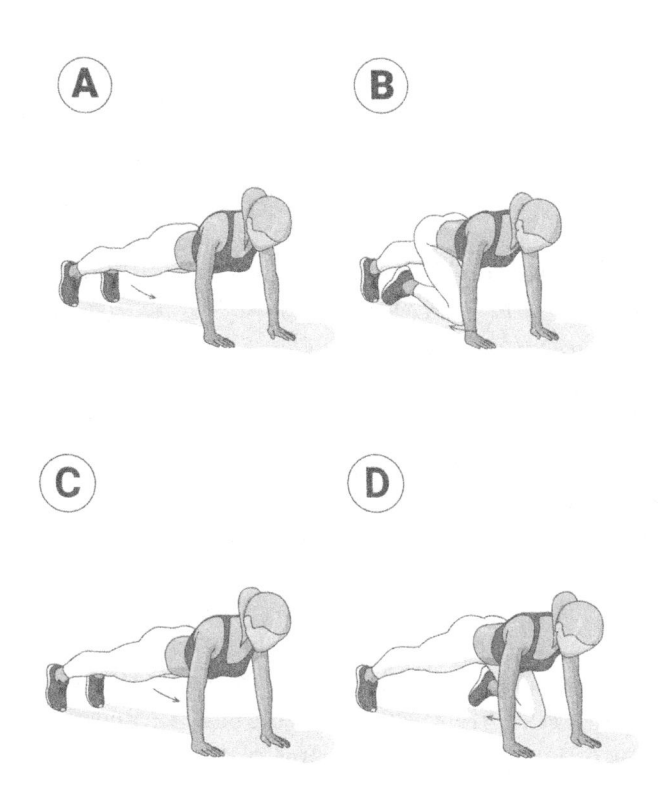

(A) (B)

(C) (D)

4 - Plank: Assume a static plank position, engaging your abdominal, leg, and arm muscles while stabilizing your core. You can choose between the two options provided.

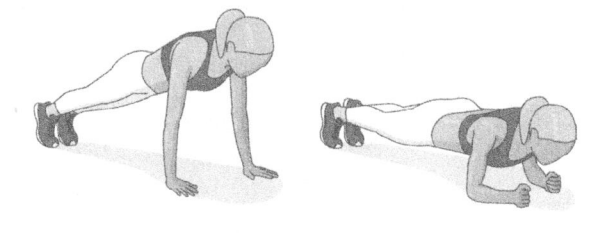

5 - Plank Walk: Engage in a walking movement while in the plank position, involving your core, arms, and legs. This exercise enhances stability and calorie burning.

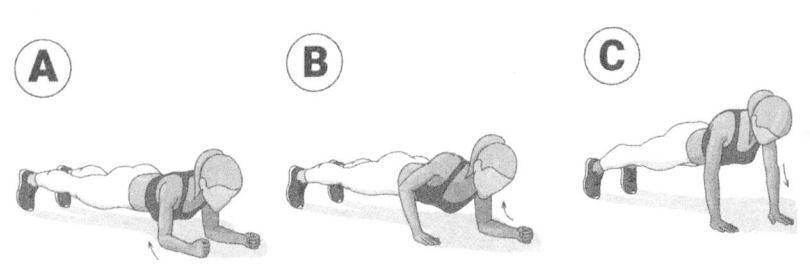

(A) (B) (C)

Remember to tailor the exercise intensity to your physical capabilities and perform a suitable warm-up before commencing your workout.

Ensure you maintain proper execution technique to prevent injuries. Be mindful of your breathing and make an effort to sustain a steady pace throughout the entire session.

Session 1 of high-intensity fat-burning exercises is a fantastic way to begin your HIIT workout journey. Experiment with the intensity levels and recovery times to discover the optimal balance and push yourself.

Always remember to listen to your body and adapt the workout to suit your capabilities.

Happy training!

Session 2: Building and Toning Muscles with Targeted Exercises

Session 2 focuses on developing and toning muscles through specific exercises. During this training phase, I emphasize precise movements that engage specific muscle groups.

Here's how I structure this session: Description: In this session, I perform a series of exercises designed to target different areas of the body, including squats, lunges, push-ups, planks, and abdominal exercises. These exercises are tailored to stimulate and strengthen muscles in a specific manner.

Timing: Each exercise is performed for 50 seconds, followed by 10 seconds of active recovery. The entire session lasts for 5 minutes.

Difficulty: Exercise difficulty can be adjusted to match your strength and fitness level. You can adapt the intensity by altering the number of repetitions or modifying the range of motion. Choose an appropriate weight or resistance based on your capabilities.

Exercise Sequence: You can follow the suggested exercise order below or customize it according to your preferences:

SHEET 1 - GOAL: DEVELOP AND TONE MUSCLES WITH SPECIFIC EXERCISES.

50" exercise - 10" active rest = 5 minutes

1 - Squat

2 - Lunges

3 - Push-ups

4 - Plank

5 - Crunches

EXERCISES AND DESCRIPTIONS:

1 - Squats: Begin by standing upright, then bend your knees and lower your body as if you were sitting on an imaginary chair. Ensure your back remains straight, and your weight is distributed evenly on your heels. Repeat this movement for the entire exercise duration.

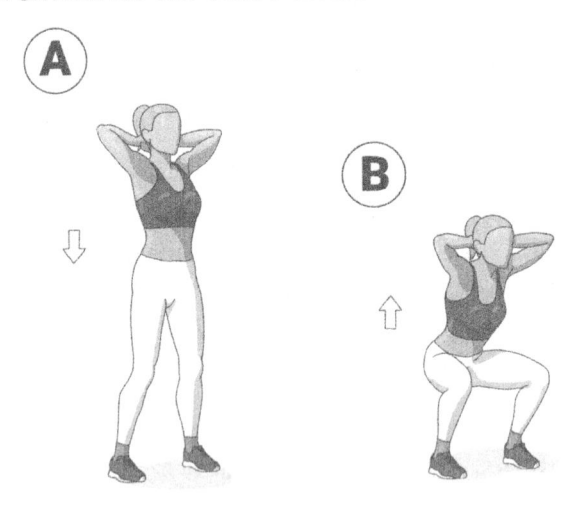

2 - Lunges: Begin standing, take a step forward with one leg, lowering your body to create a 90-degree angle with both knees. Return to standing and repeat with the other leg. Continue alternating legs for the entire duration of the exercise.

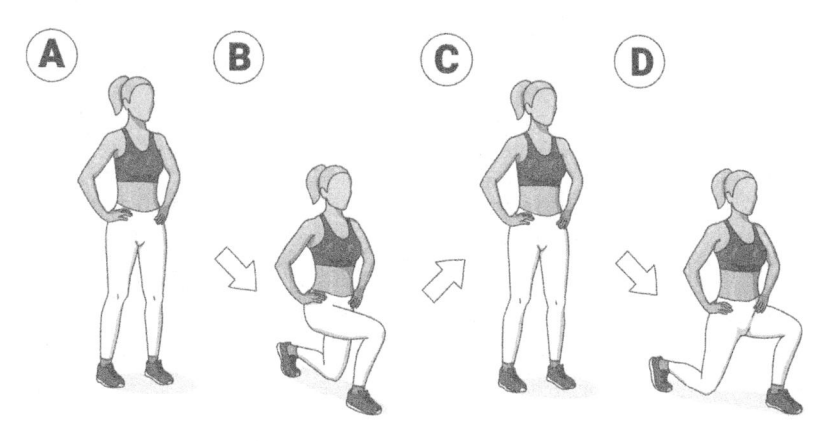

3 - Push-ups: Start in a plank position, lower your body by bending your arms, and push back up to a plank position. Ensure good posture and control throughout the movement. Repeat the movement for the entire duration of the exercise.

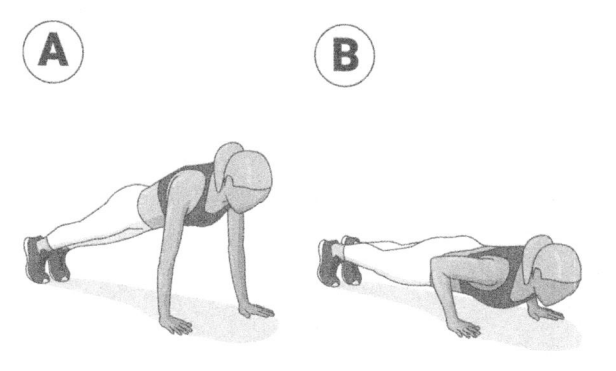

4 - Plank: Assume a static plank position, engaging your abdominal, leg, and arm muscles while stabilizing your core. You can choose between the two options provided.

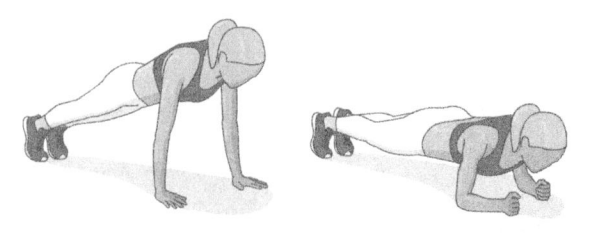

5 - Crunches (Abdominals): You can choose the type of abdominal exercise you prefer, such as crunches, sit-ups, or bicycle crunches. Focus on engaging your abdominal muscles and maintain proper form.

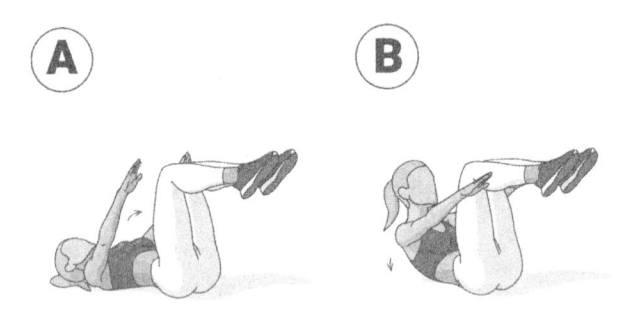

(A) (B)

Remember to adjust the exercise intensity to your physical abilities and perform a proper warm-up before starting your workout.

SHEET 2 - GOAL: DEVELOP AND TONE MUSCLES WITH SPECIFIC EXERCISES.

50" exercise - 10" active rest = 5 minutes

1 - Burpees

2 - Mountain Climbers

3 - Plank Jack with Push-up

4 - Plank

5 - Push-up with Mountain Climber

EXERCISES AND DESCRIPTIONS:

1 - Burpees: Start in a standing position. Perform a push-up, then jump into a squat position, and finally, leap up with arms raised overhead. Repeat the movement throughout the exercise duration.

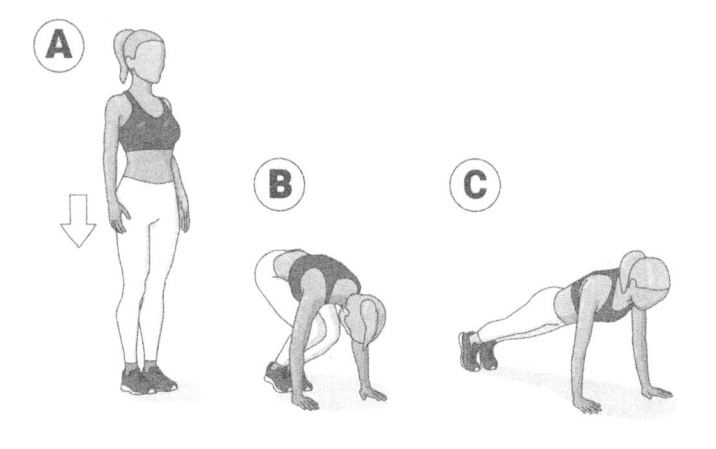

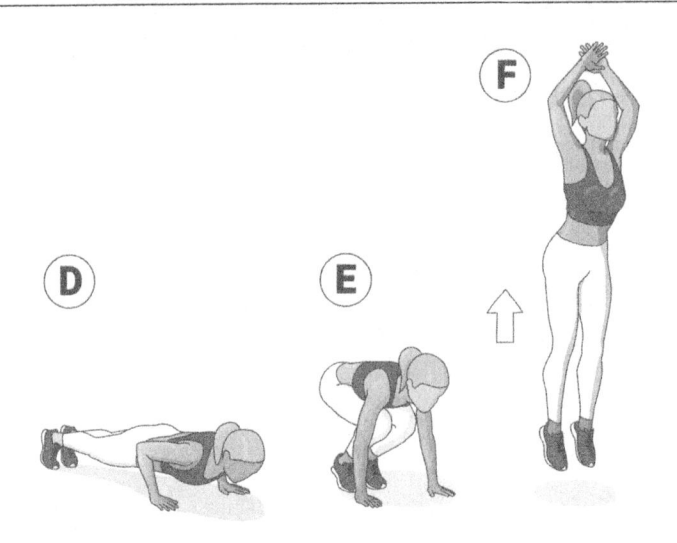

2 - Mountain Climbers: Start in a plank position, then quickly and controlledly bring the knees alternately towards the chest. Keep alternating legs throughout the exercise duration.

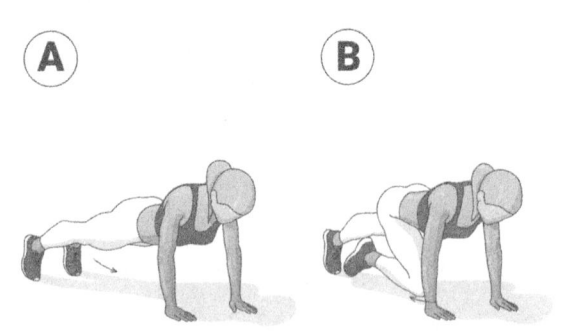

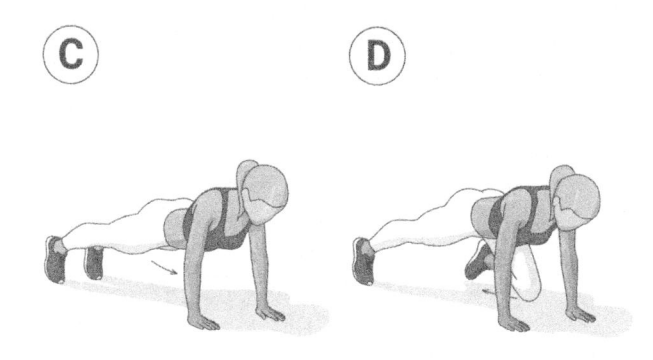

3 - Plank Jack with Push-up: Position yourself in a plank position, with arms extended and the body in a straight line. Jump your feet apart, then perform a push-up. Repeat the movement smoothly for the entire duration of the exercise.

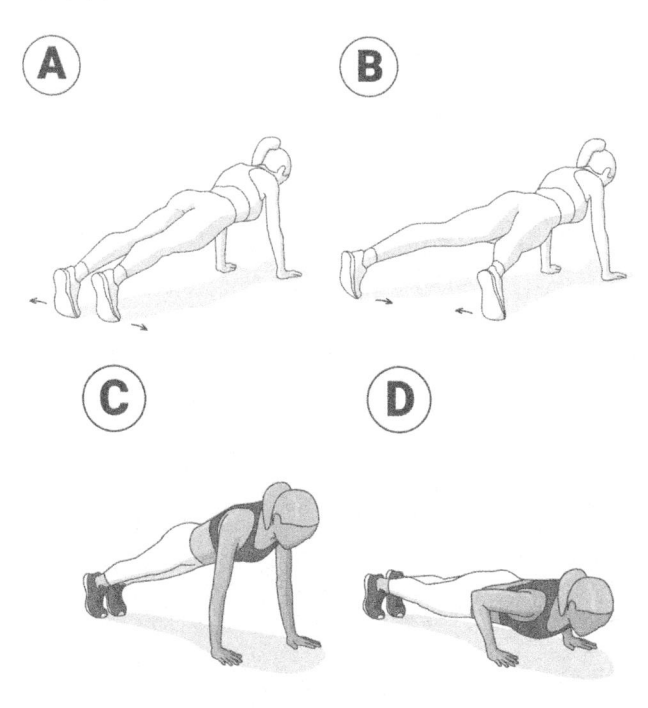

4 - Plank: Assume a static plank position, engaging your abdominal, leg, and arm muscles while stabilizing your core. You can choose between the two options provided.

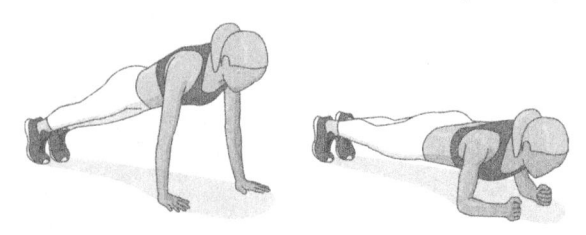

5 - Push-up with Mountain Climber: Begin with a push-up on the ground, then, as you return to the plank position, alternately bring your right knee and left knee towards your chest at a brisk pace. Continue this leg alternation throughout the exercise.

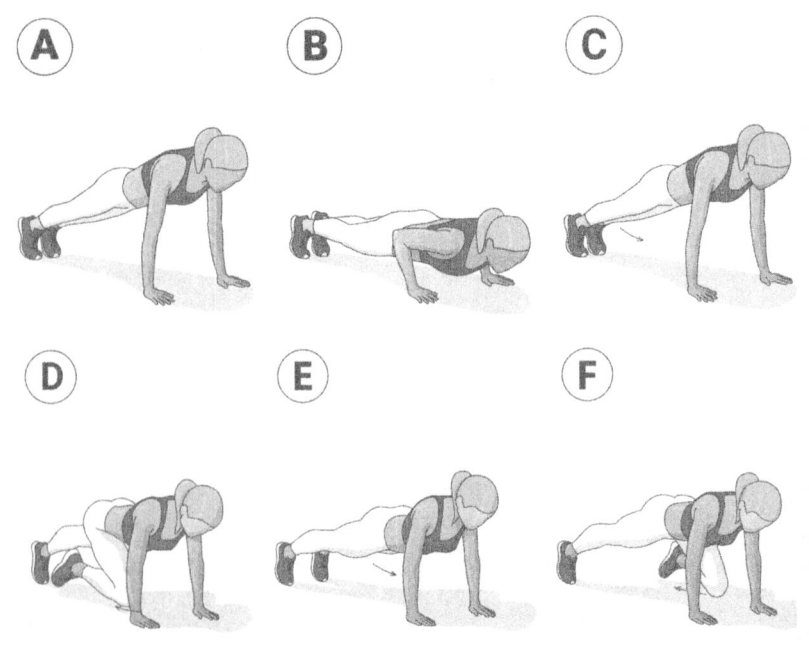

(A) (B) (C)

(D) (E) (F)

Remember to adjust the exercise intensity to your physical abilities and perform a proper warm-up before starting your workout.

SHEET 3 - GOAL: DEVELOP AND TONE MUSCLES WITH SPECIFIC EXERCISES.

50" exercise - 10" active rest = 5 minutes

1 - Jump Squats

2 - Lunges to Knee Drive

3 - Plank Jack with Push-up

4 - Traditional Lunges

5 - Knee to Elbow

EXERCISES AND DESCRIPTIONS:

1 - Jump Squats: Perform a squat followed by a high jump. This activates leg, glute, and abdominal muscles, boosting endurance and calorie burn.

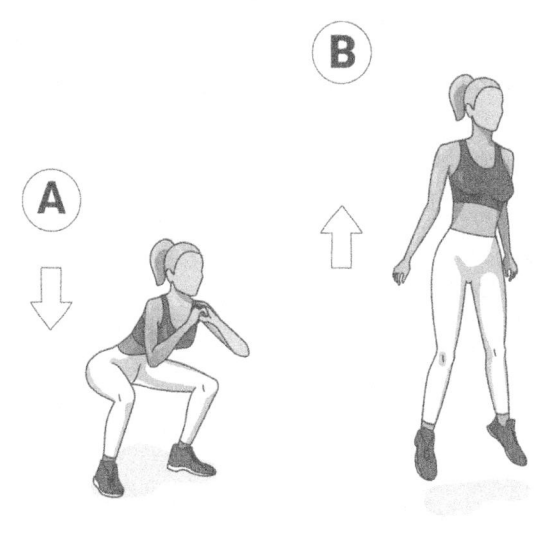

2 - Lunges to Knee Drive: Start standing with feet hip-width apart. Take a step forward with your right foot, bending your knees to lower towards the floor. Then, push your body upward, focusing on the front leg, and bring your left knee towards your chest during the upward push. Alternate sides by taking a step forward with your left foot and bringing your right knee towards your chest during the upward push.

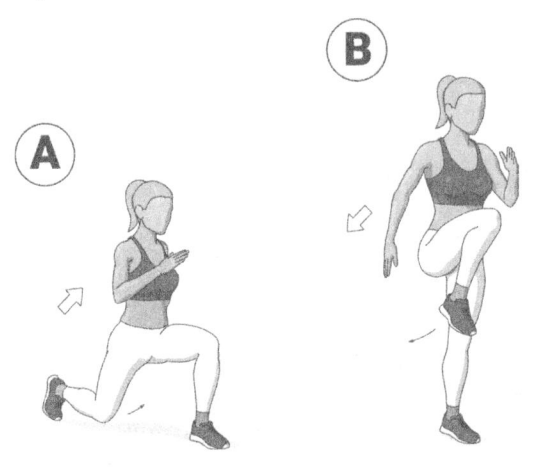

3 - Plank Jack with Push-up: Position yourself in a plank position, with arms extended and the body in a straight line. Jump your feet apart, then perform a push-up. Repeat the movement smoothly for the entire duration of the exercise.

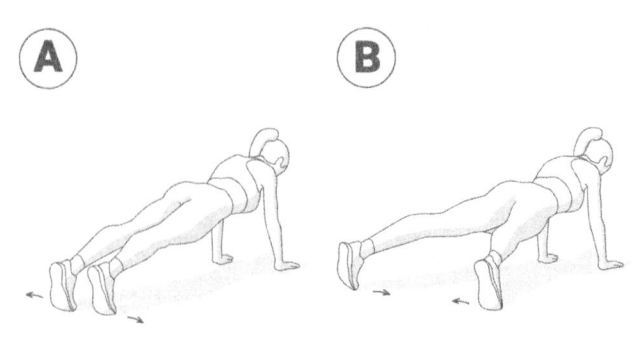

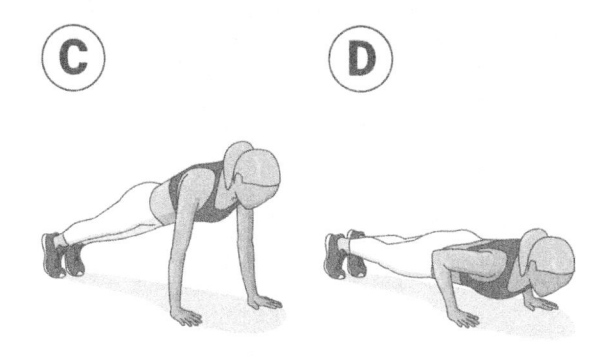

4 - Traditional Lunges: Perform classic lunges, engaging the leg and glute muscles while increasing your heart rate and burning calories.

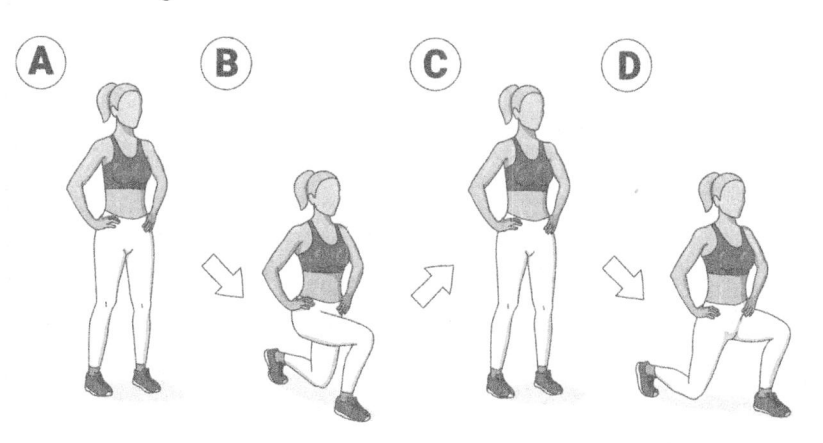

5 - Knee to Elbow: Assume a plank position while bringing your knee close to your elbow. This exercise engages your oblique abdominal muscles and core, promoting fat burning.

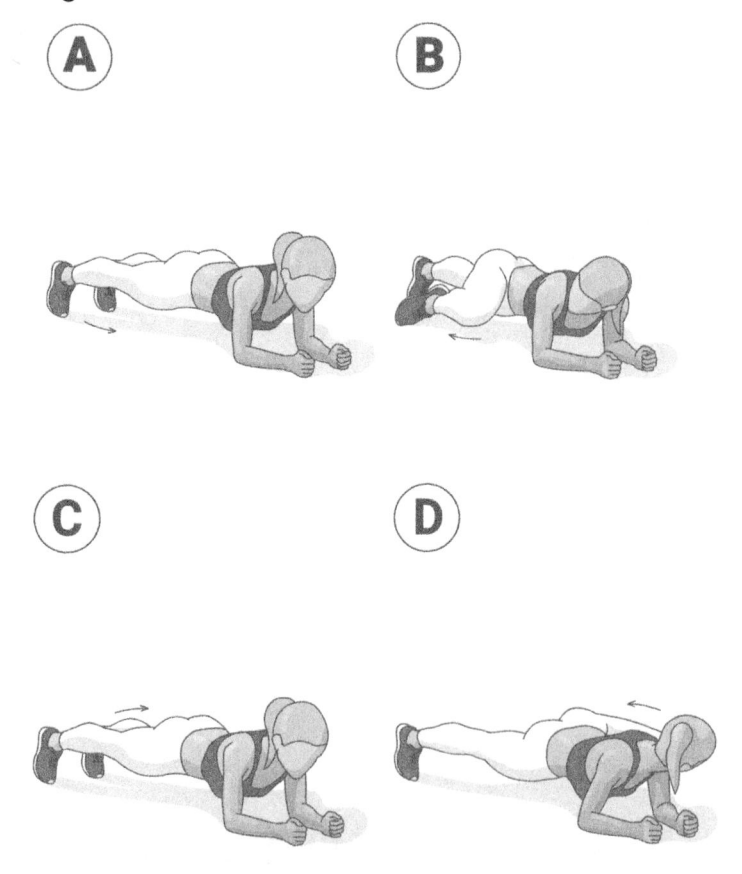

(A) (B)

(C) (D)

Remember to adjust the intensity of the exercises to your physical abilities and perform a proper warm-up before starting the workout.

SHEET 4 - GOAL: DEVELOP AND TONE MUSCLES WITH SPECIFIC EXERCISES.

50" exercise - 10" active rest = 5 minutes

1 - Jumping Jacks

2 - Abdominals (Crunches)

3 - High Knees

4 - Plank Shoulder Taps

5 - Swimmer

EXERCISES AND DESCRIPTIONS:

1 - Jumping Jacks: Begin in a standing position with legs together and arms down at the sides. Then jump, spreading the legs laterally and raising the arms overhead. Return to the starting position and repeat the movement for the entire exercise duration.

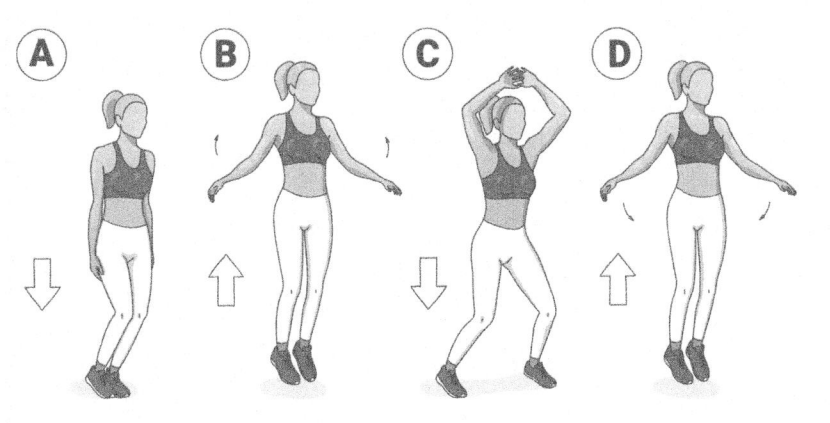

2 - Crunches (Abdominals): You can choose the type of abdominal exercise you prefer, such as crunches, sit-ups, or bicycle crunches. Focus on engaging your abdominal muscles and maintain proper form.

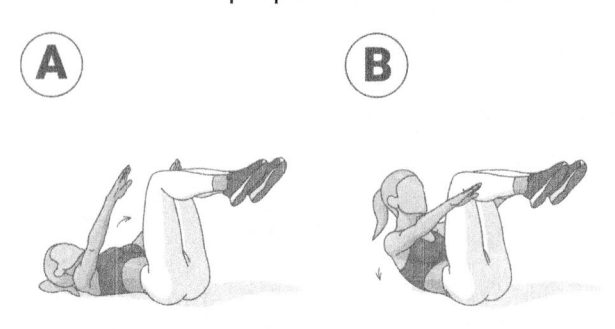

3 - High Knees: Begin in a standing position with arms relaxed at the sides. Take a step forward, raising one knee high towards the chest while simultaneously lifting the opposite arm upward. Quickly alternate legs, maintaining a fast pace and aiming to lift the knees as high as possible. This exercise engages the abs, legs, and improves cardiovascular endurance.

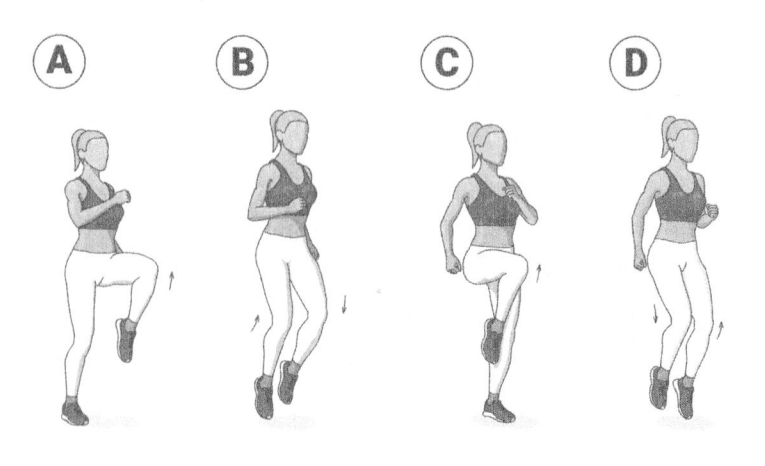

4 - Plank Shoulder Taps: Assume a plank position and alternate tapping your shoulders. This targets your abs, oblique abdominals, and activates the shoulder stabilizers.

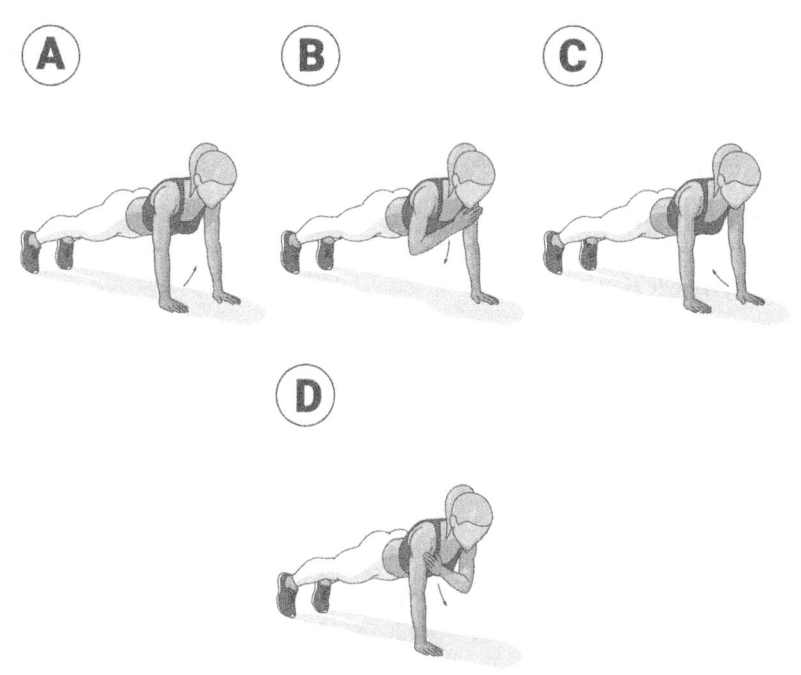

(A) (B) (C)

(D)

5 - Swimmer: This exercise mimics the motions of swimming and engages your core, arms, and legs. It promotes fat burning and increases muscle endurance.

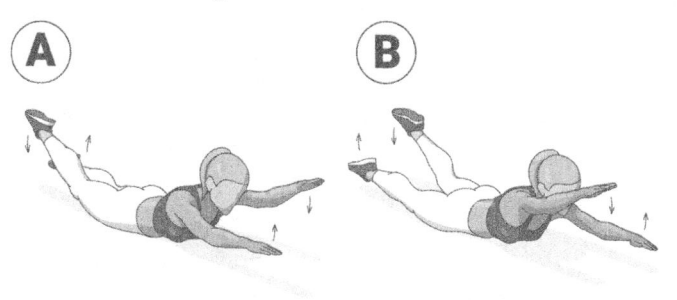

(A) (B)

Remember to adjust the intensity of the exercises to your

physical abilities and to perform a proper warm-up before starting your workout.

SHEET 5 - GOAL: DEVELOP AND TONE MUSCLES WITH SPECIFIC EXERCISES.

50" exercise - 10" active rest = 5 minutes

1 - Push-ups

2 - Flutter Kicks

3 - Plank

4 - Knee to Elbow

5 - Plank Walk

EXERCISES AND DESCRIPTIONS:

1 - Push-ups: Start in a plank position, lower your body by bending your arms, and push back up to a plank position. Ensure good posture and control throughout the movement. Repeat the movement for the entire duration of the exercise.

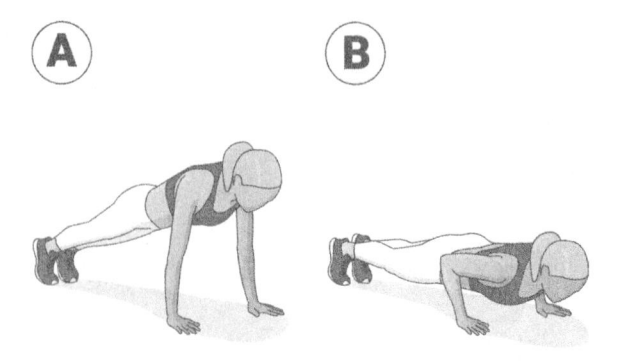

2 - Flutter Kicks: Lie on your back and lift your legs in a fluttering motion. This targets your lower abdominal muscles, leg muscles, and helps burn calories.

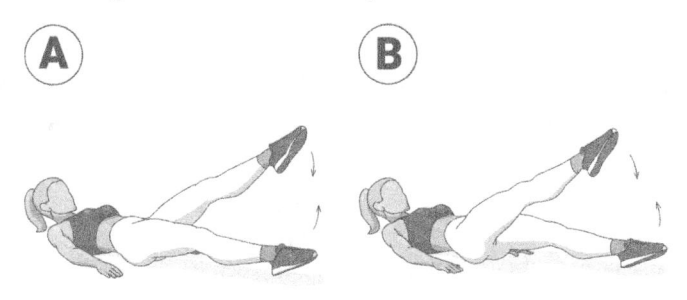

(A) (B)

3 - Plank: Assume a static plank position, engaging your abdominal, leg, and arm muscles while stabilizing your core. You can choose between the two options provided.

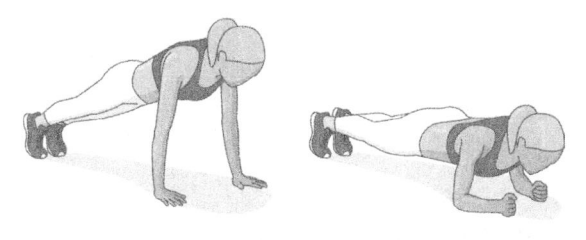

4 - Knee to Elbow: Assume a plank position while bringing your knee close to your elbow. This exercise engages your oblique abdominal muscles and core, promoting fat burning.

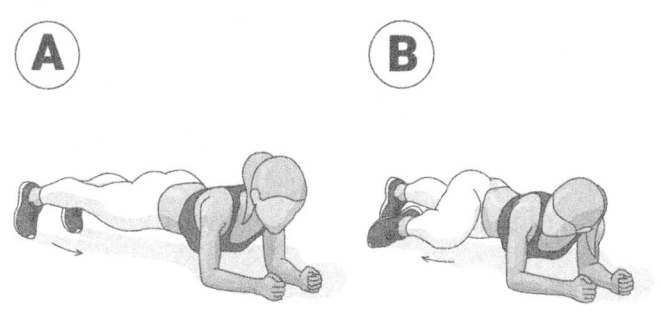

(A) (B)

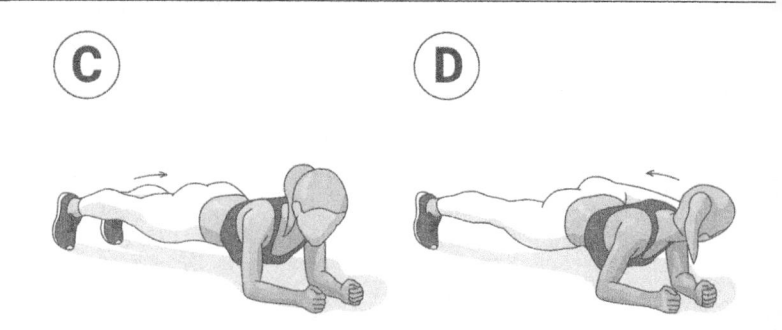

5 - Plank Walk: Engage in a walking movement while in the plank position, involving your core, arms, and legs. This exercise enhances stability and calorie burning.

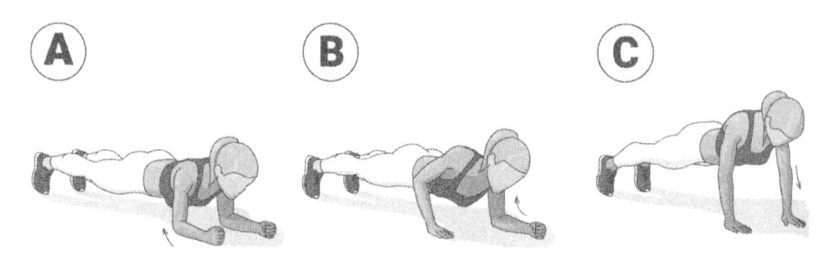

Remember to adjust the intensity of the exercises to your physical capabilities and perform a proper warm-up before starting the workout.

Remember to maintain good exercise technique and adapt the intensity according to your abilities. The goal is to work on the muscles in a targeted manner, feeling fatigue but without overdoing it.

Session 2 of muscle development and toning with specific exercises will help you strengthen and define your body. Customize the exercises to meet your needs and enjoy the process of building strength and muscle tone.

Session 3: Comprehensive Circuits for Total Body Engagement

In session 3, my focus shifts to comprehensive circuits designed to engage all muscle groups across the body. This session presents an opportunity to put my overall endurance and strength to the test. Here's how I structure this workout:

Description: During this session, I perform a series of exercises that simultaneously target different muscle groups. These include exercises like squat thrusts, plank with mountain climbers, and lunges with lateral raises. These full-body circuits enable me to work synergistically on all muscle groups.

Timing: Each exercise is executed for 40 seconds, followed by 20 seconds of active recovery. The entire circuit takes 5 minutes to complete.

Difficulty: The level of difficulty can be adjusted based on your individual strength and training experience. You have the flexibility to increase or decrease intensity by modifying weights or resistance levels. Choose a difficulty level that challenges you while allowing you to maintain proper exercise technique.

Exercise Sequence: You can adhere to the suggested exercise order below or customize it according to your preferences:

Remember to tailor the exercise intensity to your personal physical capabilities and ensure you perform a suitable warm-up prior to commencing your workout.

SHEET 1 - GOAL: FULL BODY CIRCUIT TO ENGAGE ALL MUSCLES.

40" exercise - 20" active rest = 5 minutes

1 - Jump Squat

2 - Plank Walk

3 - Lunges

4 - Push-up with Mountain Climber

5 - Jumping Lunges

EXERCISES AND DESCRIPTIONS:

1 - Jump Squat: Start in a standing position, then jump up and land in a squat position. Jump again to return to the standing position and repeat the movement throughout the exercise duration.

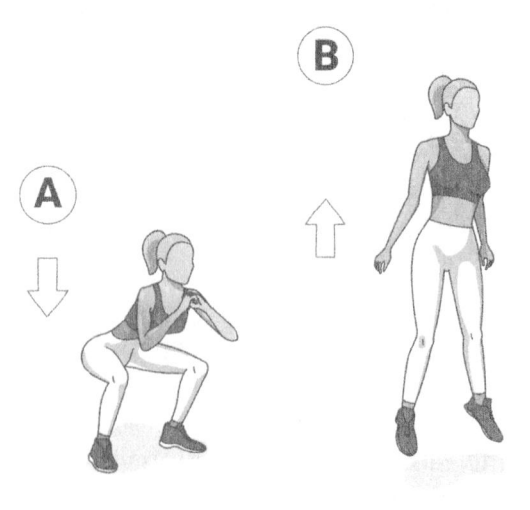

2 - Plank Walk: Engage in a walking movement while in the plank position, involving your core, arms, and legs. This exercise enhances stability and calorie burning.

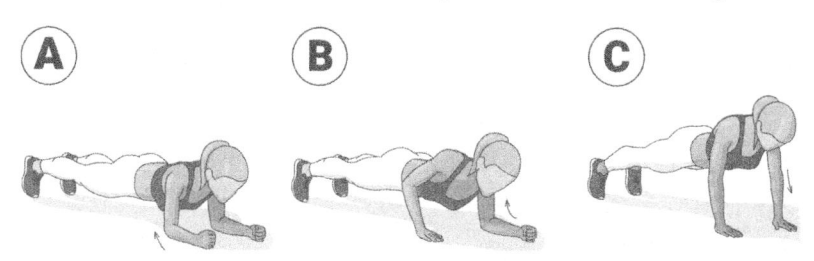

Ⓐ **Ⓑ** **Ⓒ**

3 - Lunges: Begin standing, take a step forward with one leg, lowering your body to create a 90-degree angle with both knees. Return to standing and repeat with the other leg. Continue alternating legs for the entire duration of the exercise.

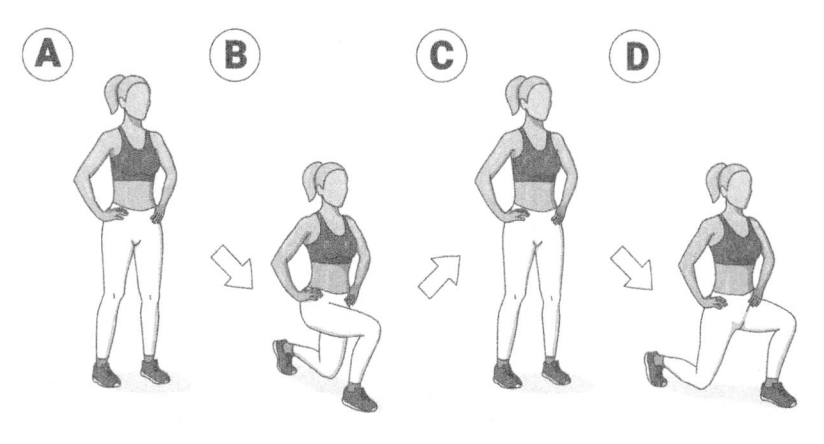

Ⓐ **Ⓑ** **Ⓒ** **Ⓓ**

4 - Push-up with Mountain Climber: Begin with a push-up on the ground, then, as you return to the plank position, alternately bring your right knee and left knee towards your chest at a brisk pace. Continue this leg alternation throughout the exercise.

→

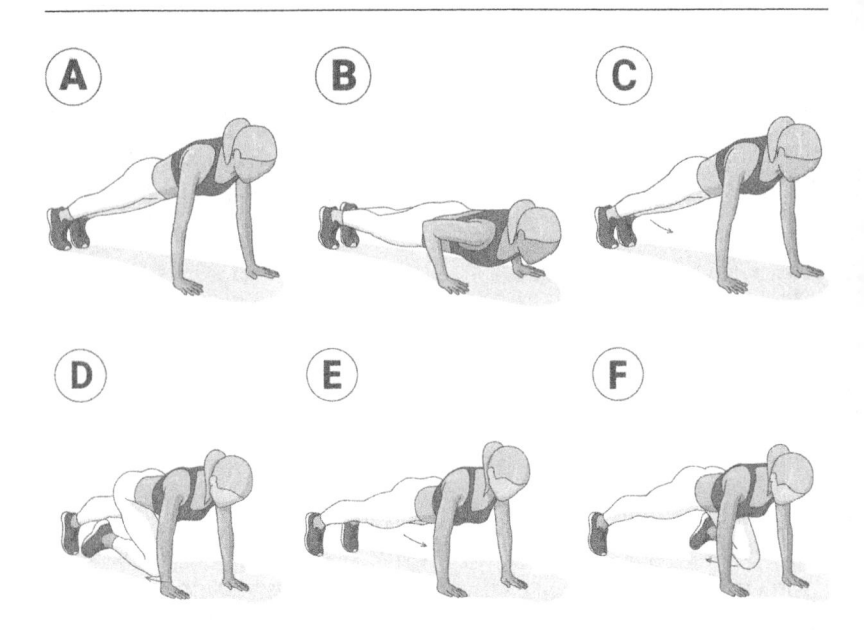

5 - Jumping Lunges: Start in a standing position with one foot forward and the other back in a lunge position. Jump, switching the positions of the legs, so that the foot that was forward is now back, and vice versa. Keep switching legs with a fast and controlled jump.

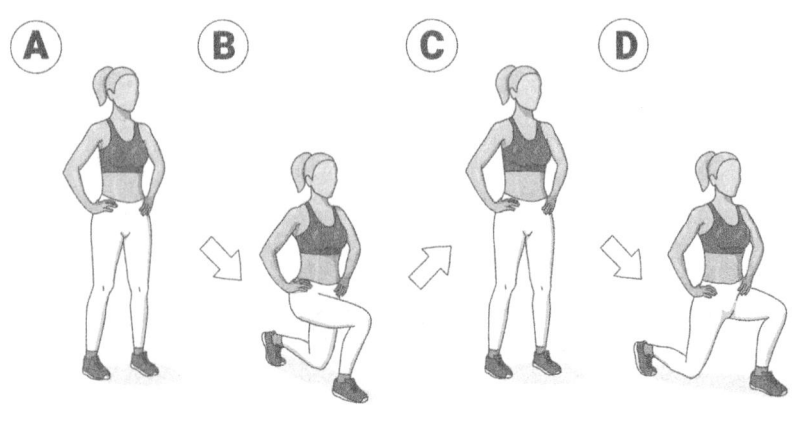

Remember to adjust the intensity of the exercises to your physical capabilities and perform a proper warm-up before

starting your workout.

SHEET 2 - GOAL: FULL-BODY CIRCUITS TO ENGAGE ALL MUSCLES.

40" exercise - 20" active rest = 5 minutes

1 - Burpees

2 - Abdominal Crunches

3 - High Knees

4 - Jump Squats

5 - Jumping Jacks

Exercises and Descriptions:

1 - Burpees: Start in a standing position. Perform a push-up, then jump into a squat position, and finally, leap up with arms raised overhead. Repeat the movement throughout the exercise duration.

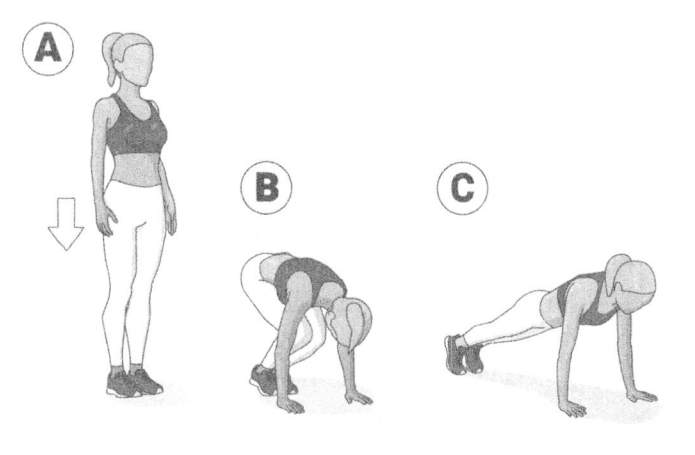

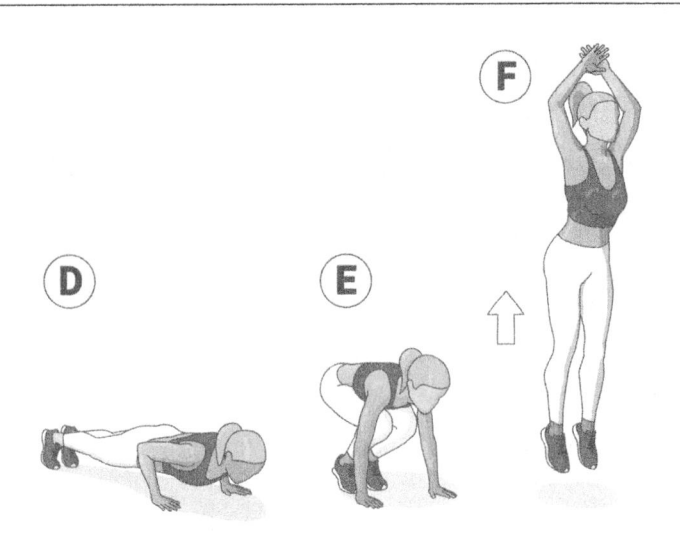

2 - Abdominal Crunches: You can choose the type of crunches you prefer, such as regular crunches, sit-ups, or bicycle crunches. Focus on engaging the abdominal muscles and maintain good form.

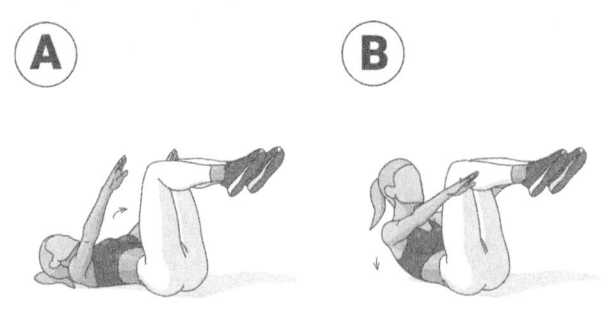

3 - High Knees: Begin in a standing position with arms relaxed at the sides. Take a step forward, raising one knee high towards the chest while simultaneously lifting the opposite arm upward. Quickly alternate legs, maintaining a fast pace and aiming to lift the knees as high as possible. This exercise engages the abs, legs, and improves cardiovascular endurance.

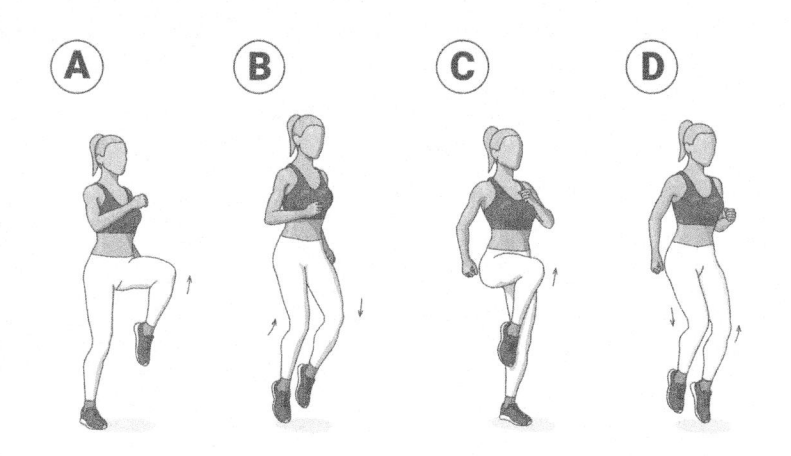

4 - Jump Squats: Perform a squat followed by a high jump. This activates leg, glute, and abdominal muscles, boosting endurance and calorie burn.

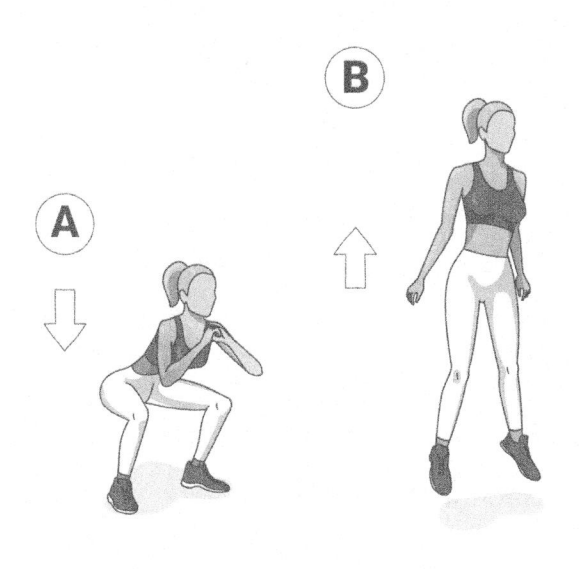

5 - Jumping Jacks: Begin in a standing position with legs together and arms down at the sides. Then jump, spreading the legs laterally and raising the arms overhead. Return to the starting position and repeat the movement for the entire exercise duration.

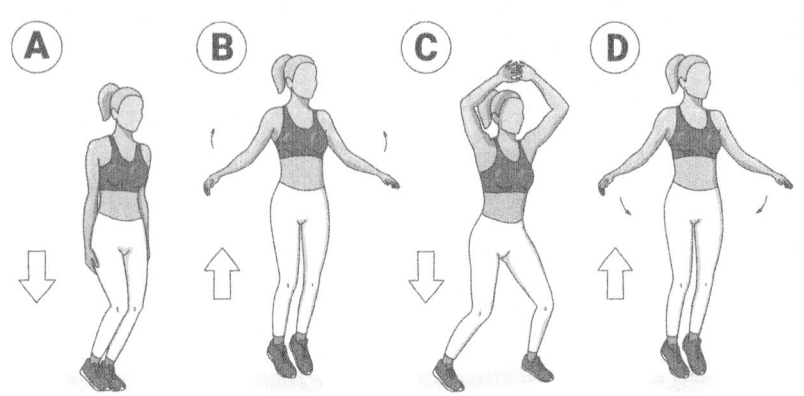

Remember to adjust the exercise intensity to your physical abilities and perform a proper warm-up before starting your workout.

SHEET 3 - GOAL: FULL-BODY CIRCUITS TO ENGAGE ALL MUSCLES.

40" exercise - 20" active rest = 5 minutes

1 - Lunges to Knee Drive

2 - Mountain Climbers

3 - Plank Jack with Push-up

4 - Plank

5 - Squat

EXERCISES AND DESCRIPTIONS:

1 - Lunges to Knee Drive: Start standing with feet hip-width apart. Take a step forward with your right foot, bending your knees to lower towards the floor. Then, push your body upward, focusing on the front leg, and bring your left knee towards your chest during the upward push. Alternate sides by taking a step forward with your left foot and bringing your right knee towards your chest during the upward push.

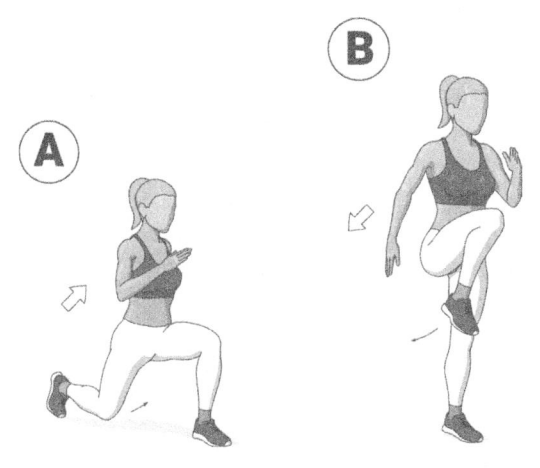

2 - Mountain Climbers: Start in a plank position, then quickly and controlledly bring the knees alternately towards the chest. Keep alternating legs throughout the exercise duration.

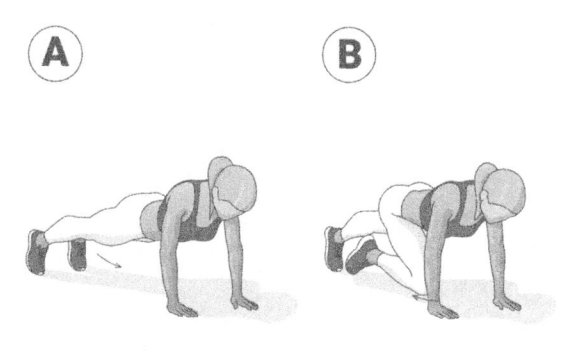

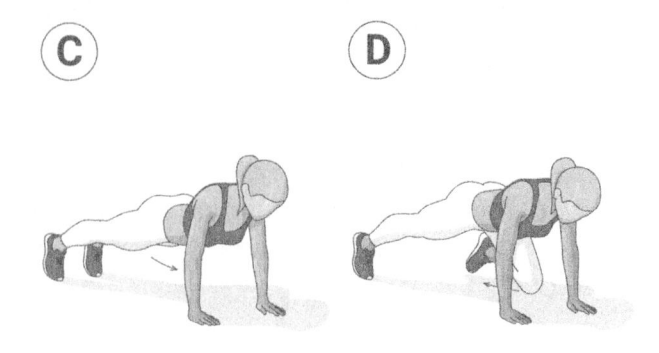

3 - Plank Jack with Push-up: Position yourself in a plank position, with arms extended and the body in a straight line. Jump your feet apart, then perform a push-up. Repeat the movement smoothly for the entire duration of the exercise.

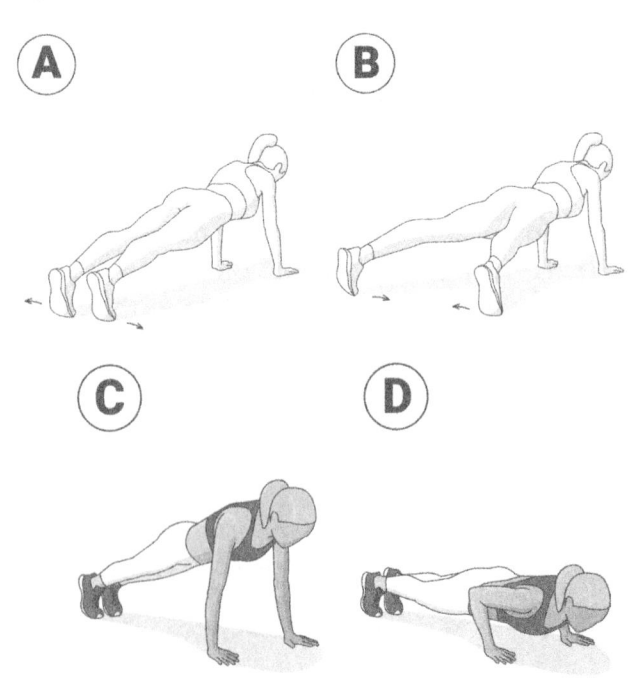

4 - Plank: Assume a static plank position, engaging your abdominal, leg, and arm muscles while stabilizing your core. You can choose between the two options provided.

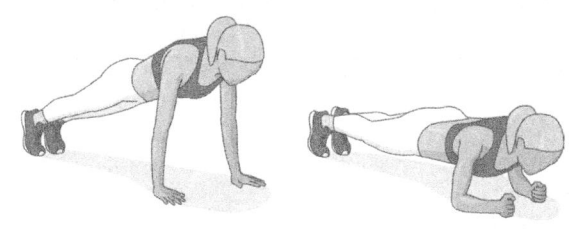

5 - Squats: Begin by standing upright, then bend your knees and lower your body as if you were sitting on an imaginary chair. Ensure your back remains straight, and your weight is distributed evenly on your heels. Repeat this movement for the entire exercise duration.

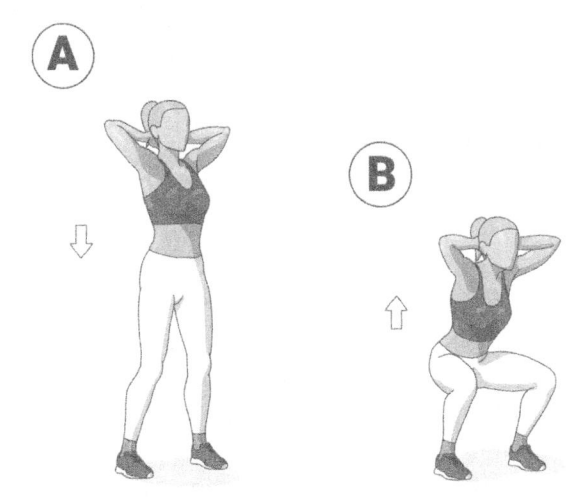

Remember to adjust the intensity of the exercises to your physical abilities and perform a proper warm-up before starting your workout.

SHEET 4 - GOAL: FULL-BODY CIRCUITS TO ENGAGE ALL MUSCLES.

40" exercise - 20" active rest = 5 minutes

1 - Push-up with mountain climber

2 - Push-ups

3 - Squat

4 - Jumping Lunges

5 - Plank Shoulder Taps

EXERCISES AND DESCRIPTIONS:

1 - Push-up with Mountain Climber: Begin with a push-up on the ground, then, as you return to the plank position, alternately bring your right knee and left knee towards your chest at a brisk pace. Continue this leg alternation throughout the exercise.

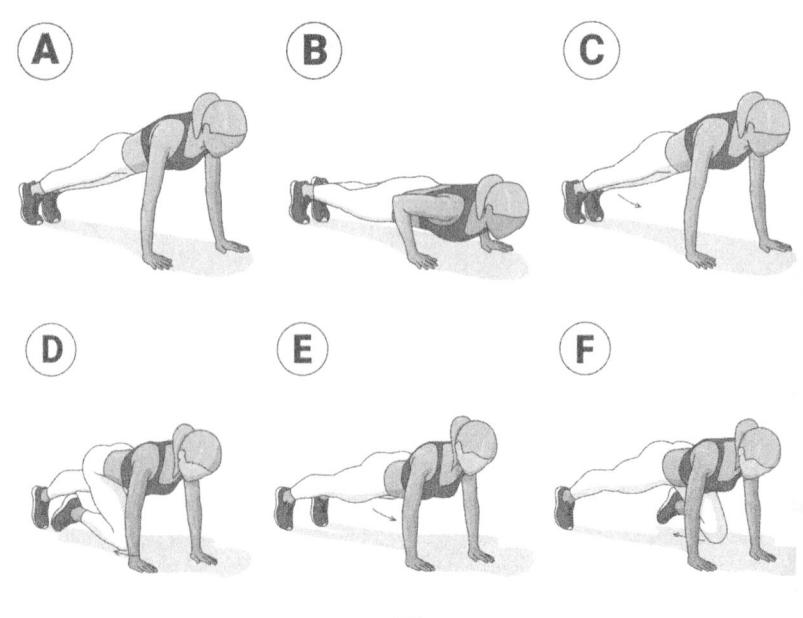

2 - Push-ups: Start in a plank position, lower your body by bending your arms, and push back up to a plank position. Ensure good posture and control throughout the movement. Repeat the movement for the entire duration of the exercise.

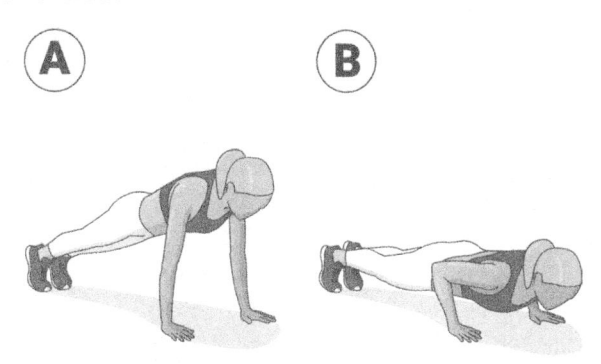

3 - Squats: Begin by standing upright, then bend your knees and lower your body as if you were sitting on an imaginary chair. Ensure your back remains straight, and your weight is distributed evenly on your heels. Repeat this movement for the entire exercise duration.

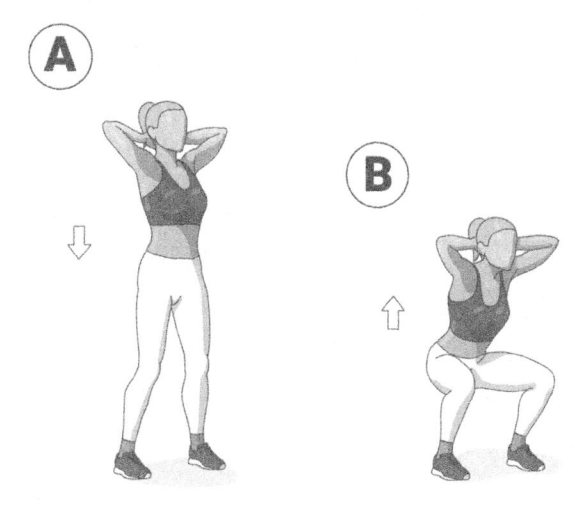

4 - Jumping Lunges: Start in a standing position with one foot forward and the other back in a lunge position. Jump, switching the positions of the legs, so that the foot that was forward is now back, and vice versa. Keep switching legs with a fast and controlled jump.

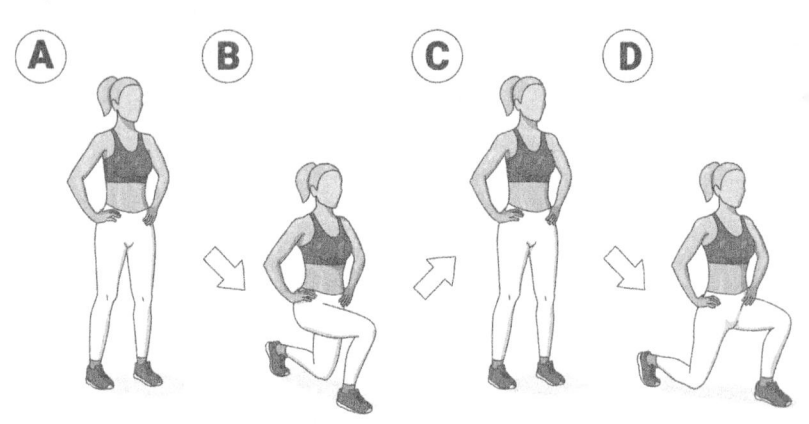

5 - Plank Shoulder Taps: Assume a plank position and alternate tapping your shoulders. This targets your abs, oblique abdominals, and activates the shoulder stabilizers.

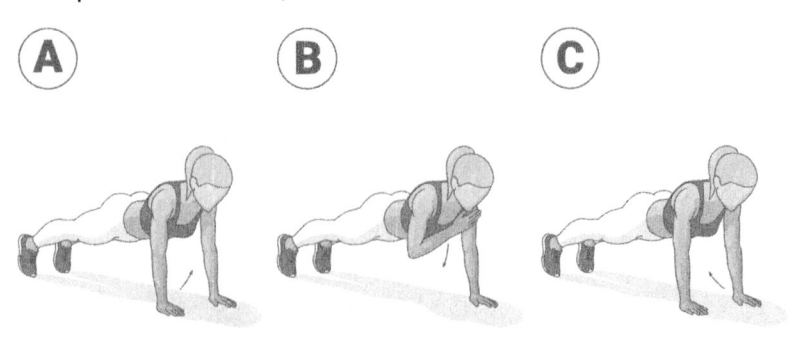

(D)

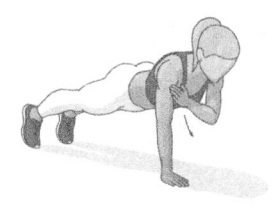

Remember to adjust the intensity of the exercises according to your physical abilities and to perform a proper warm-up before starting the workout.

SHEET 5 - OBJECTIVE: FULL-BODY CIRCUITS TO ENGAGE ALL MUSCLES.

40" exercise - 20" active rest = 5 minutes

1 - Burpees

2 - Plank Walk

3 - Jump Squats

4 - Abdominals (Crunches)

5 - Plank

EXERCISES AND DESCRIPTIONS:

1 - Burpees: Start in a standing position. Perform a push-up, then jump into a squat position, and finally, leap up with arms raised overhead. Repeat the movement throughout the exercise duration.

→

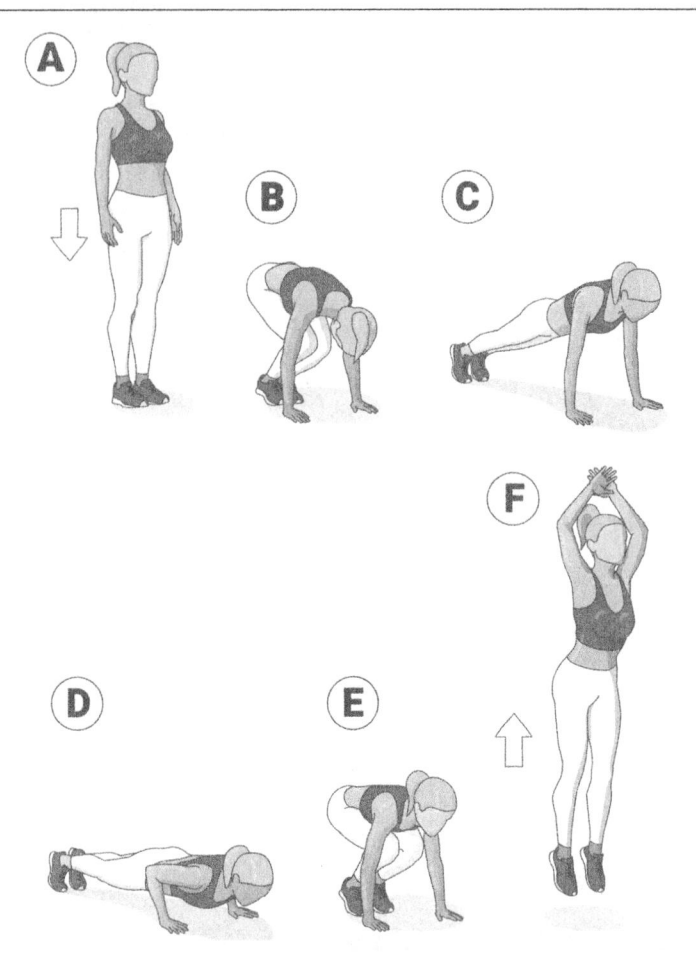

2 - Plank Walk: Engage in a walking movement while in the plank position, involving your core, arms, and legs. This exercise enhances stability and calorie burning.

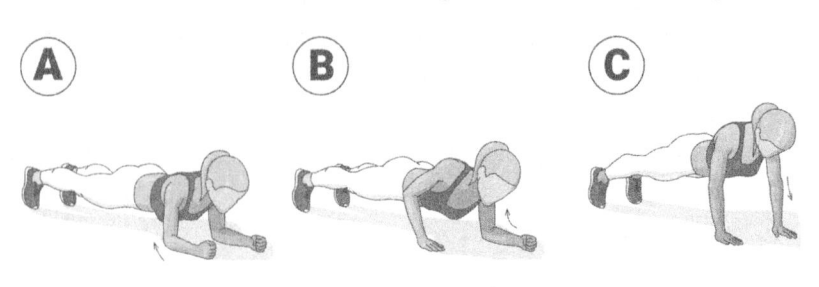

70

3 - Jump Squats: Perform a squat followed by a high jump. This activates leg, glute, and abdominal muscles, boosting endurance and calorie burn.

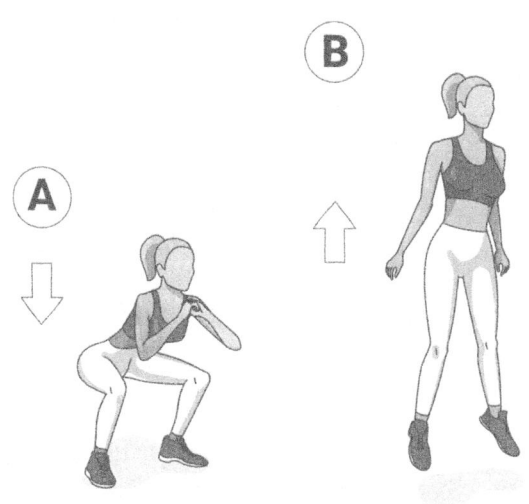

4 - Crunches (Abdominals): You can choose the type of abdominal exercise you prefer, such as crunches, sit-ups, or bicycle crunches. Focus on engaging your abdominal muscles and maintain proper form.

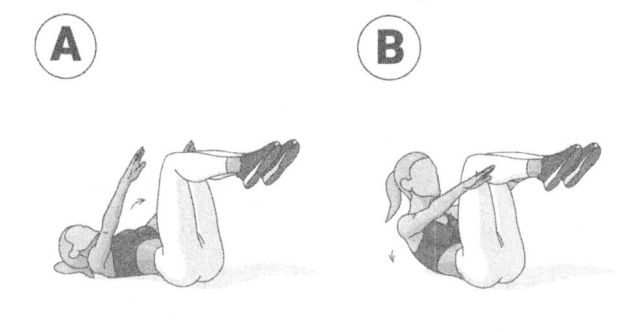

5 - Plank: Assume a static plank position, engaging your abdominal, leg, and arm muscles while stabilizing your core. You can choose between the two options provided.

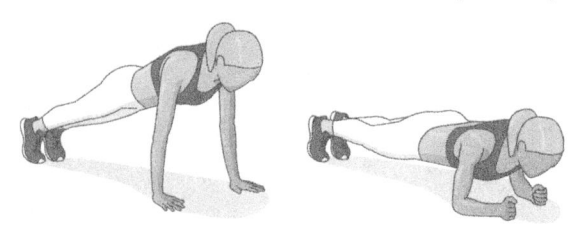

Remember to adjust the intensity of the exercises according to your physical abilities and to perform a proper warm-up before starting the workout.

At the end of this session, I feel satisfied for having engaged my whole body and worked on endurance, strength, and coordination. Remember to adjust the exercises to your abilities and to maintain good posture and breathing during execution.

Session 4: Interval Training for Full Body Muscle Work

In session 4, I dedicate myself to interval training to work on all muscle groups in my body. This type of training allows me to combine strength exercises with high-intensity cardiovascular exercises to achieve optimal results. Here's how I structure my session:

Description: During this session, I alternate between strength exercises and high-intensity cardiovascular exercises. This way, I stimulate my muscles and burn calories simultaneously, achieving a complete muscle workout and intense cardio activity.

Timing: Each exercise is performed for 45 seconds, followed by 15 seconds of active recovery. I complete the circuit of exercises in 5 minutes.

Difficulty: The difficulty of the exercises can be customized based on your abilities and fitness level. You can increase or decrease the intensity by adjusting the weight or resistance of the exercises. Choose a difficulty level that allows you to maintain good execution technique.

Exercise Order: You can follow the order of exercises proposed below or modify it according to your preferences:

SHEET 1 - OBJECTIVE: INTERVAL TRAINING FOR A FULL BODY WORKOUT.

45" exercise - 15" active rest = 5 minutes

1 - Jump Squats

2 - Push-ups

3 - Burpees

4 - Lunges

5 - Mountain Climbers

EXERCISES AND DESCRIPTIONS:

1 - Jump Squats: Perform a squat followed by a high jump. This activates leg, glute, and abdominal muscles, boosting endurance and calorie burn.

→

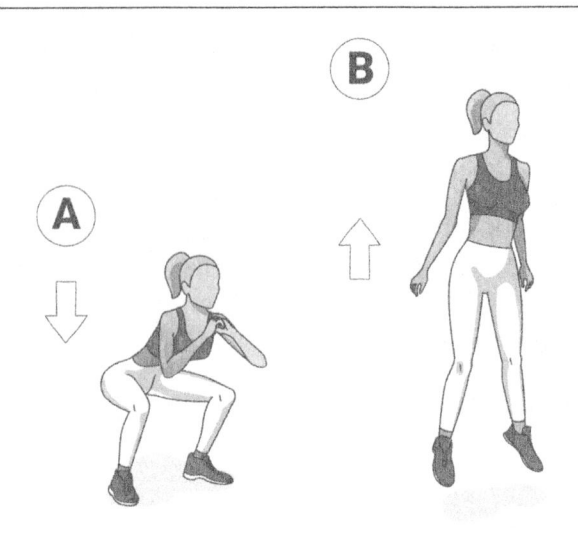

2 - Push-ups: Start in a plank position, lower your body by bending your arms, and push back up to a plank position. Ensure good posture and control throughout the movement. Repeat the movement for the entire duration of the exercise.

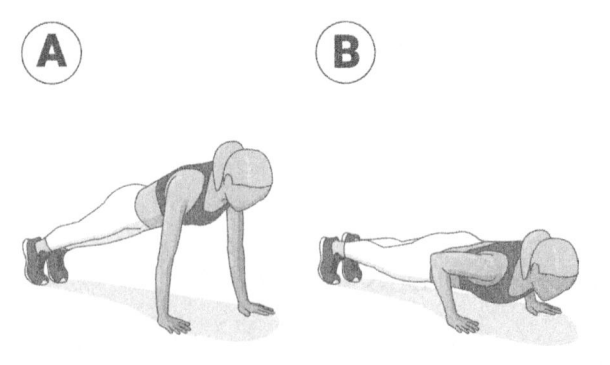

3 - Burpees: Start in a standing position. Perform a push-up, then jump into a squat position, and finally, leap up with arms raised overhead. Repeat the movement throughout the exercise duration.

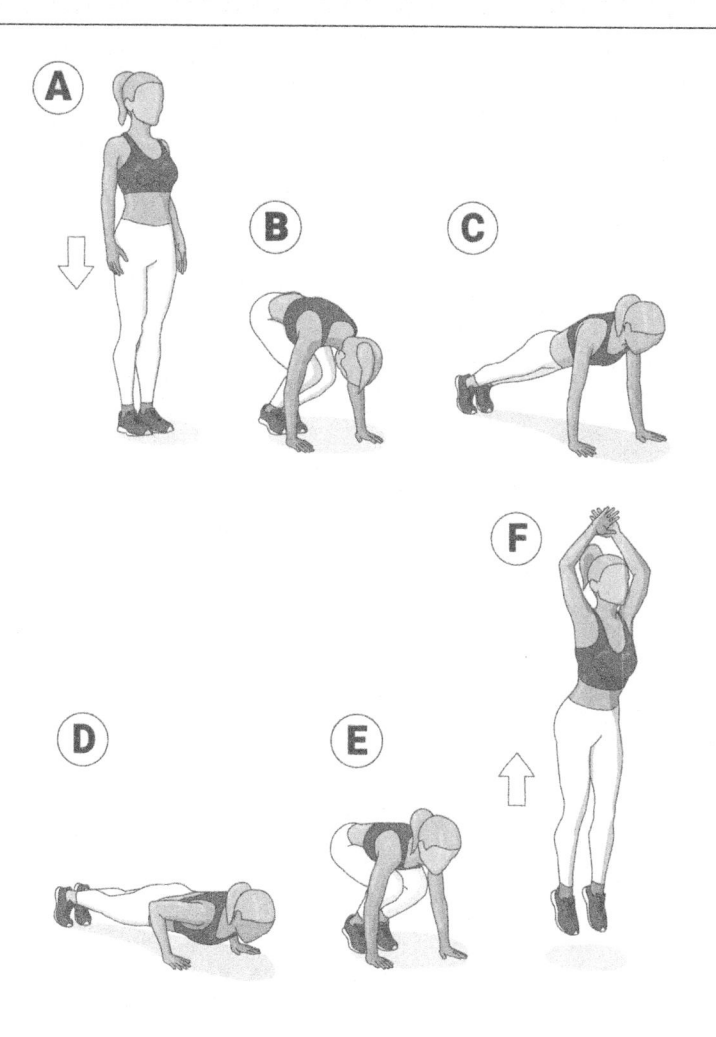

4 - Lunges: Begin standing, take a step forward with one leg, lowering your body to create a 90-degree angle with both knees. Return to standing and repeat with the other leg. Continue alternating legs for the entire duration of the exercise.

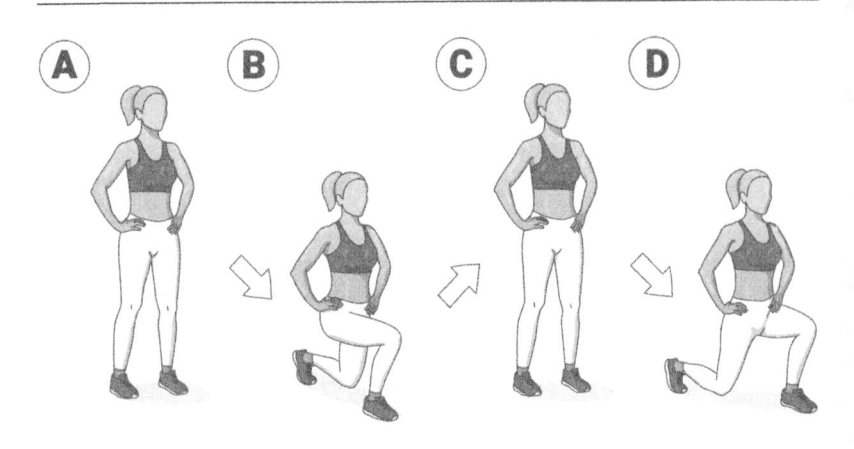

5 - Mountain Climbers: Start in a plank position, then quickly and controlledly bring the knees alternately towards the chest. Keep alternating legs throughout the exercise duration.

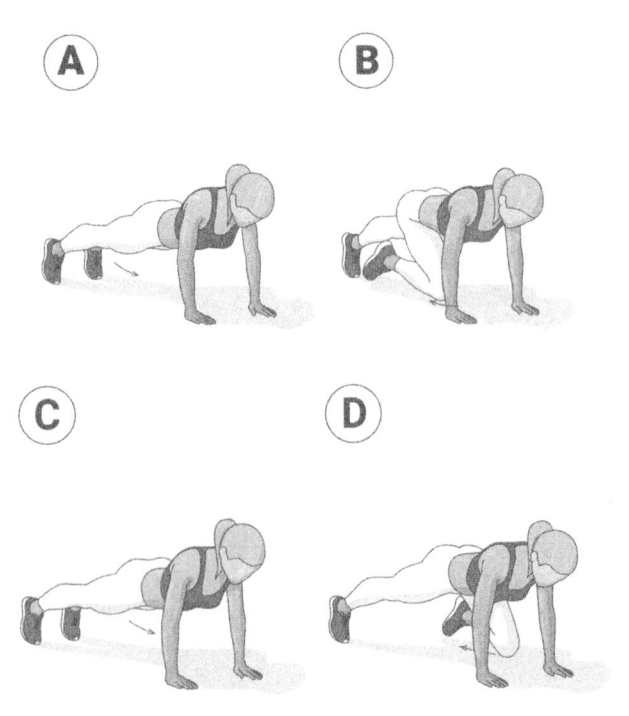

Remember to adapt the intensity of the exercises to your physical abilities and to perform a proper warm-up before starting the workout.

SHEET 2 - GOAL: INTERVAL TRAINING FOR COMPREHENSIVE MUSCLE WORK.

45" exercise - 15" active rest = 5 minutes

1 - Plank Jacks with Push-Ups

2 - Squats

3 - Abdominals (Crunches)

4 - Plank

5 - Jumping Jacks

EXERCISES AND DESCRIPTIONS:

1 - Plank Jacks with Push-up: Start in a plank position with your arms extended and your body in a straight line. Jump your feet apart, then perform a push-up. Repeat this movement smoothly for the entire exercise duration.

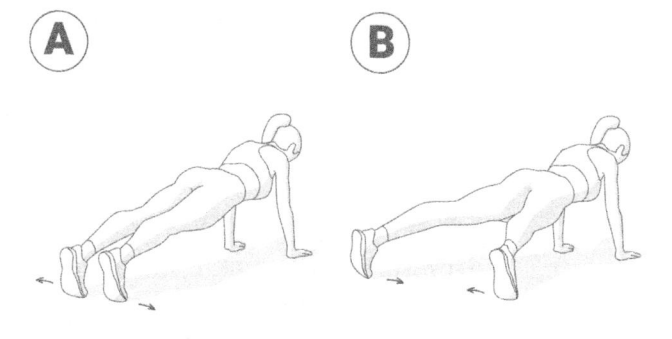

A   B

→

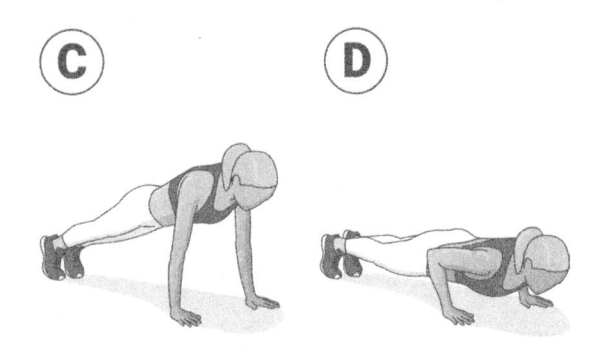

2 - Squats: Begin by standing upright, then bend your knees and lower your body as if you were sitting on an imaginary chair. Ensure your back remains straight, and your weight is distributed evenly on your heels. Repeat this movement for the entire exercise duration.

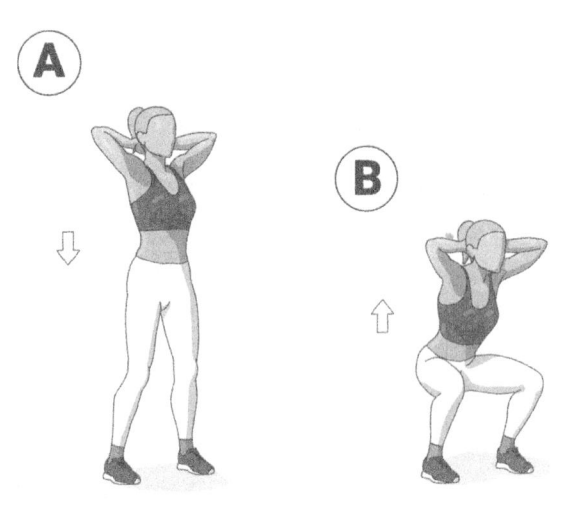

3 - Crunches (Abdominals): You can choose the type of abdominal exercise you prefer, such as crunches, sit-ups, or bicycle crunches. Focus on engaging your abdominal muscles and maintain proper form.

→

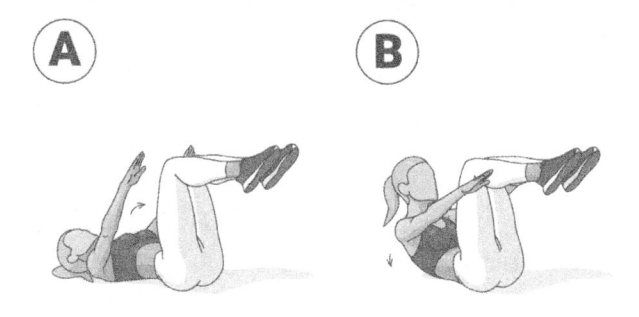

4 - Plank: Assume a static plank position, engaging your abdominal, leg, and arm muscles while stabilizing your core. You can choose between the two options provided.

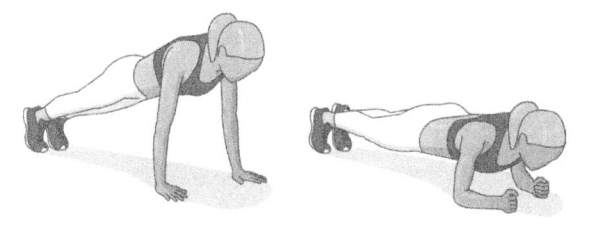

5 - Jumping Jacks: Begin in a standing position with legs together and arms down at the sides. Then jump, spreading the legs laterally and raising the arms overhead. Return to the starting position and repeat the movement for the entire exercise duration.

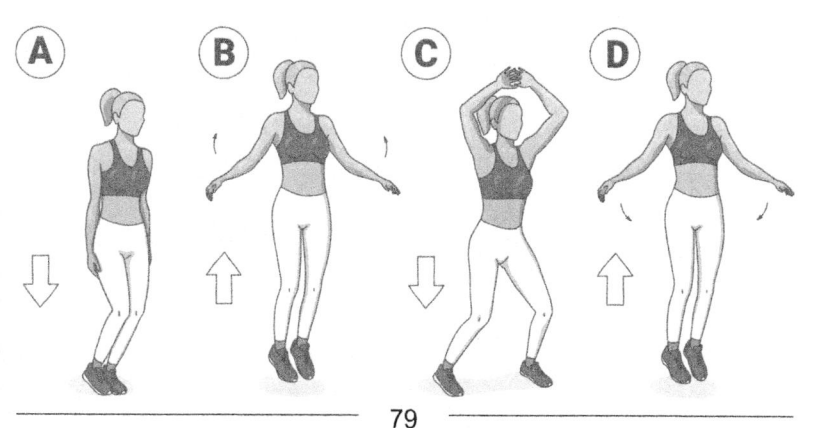

Remember to adjust the intensity of the exercises to your physical capabilities and perform a proper warm-up before starting the workout.

SHEET 3 - GOAL: INTERVAL TRAINING FOR FULL BODY MUSCLE WORK.

45" exercise - 15" active rest = 5 minutes

1 - Push-up with Mountain Climber

2 - Lunges to Knee Drive

3 - Burpees

4 - Plank Shoulder Taps

5 - High Knees

EXERCISES AND DESCRIPTIONS:

1 - Push-up with Mountain Climber: Begin with a push-up on the ground, then, as you return to the plank position, alternately bring your right knee and left knee towards your chest at a brisk pace. Continue this leg alternation throughout the exercise.

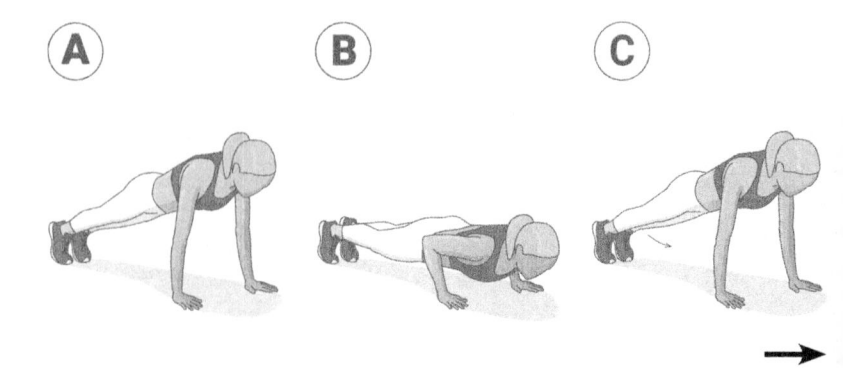

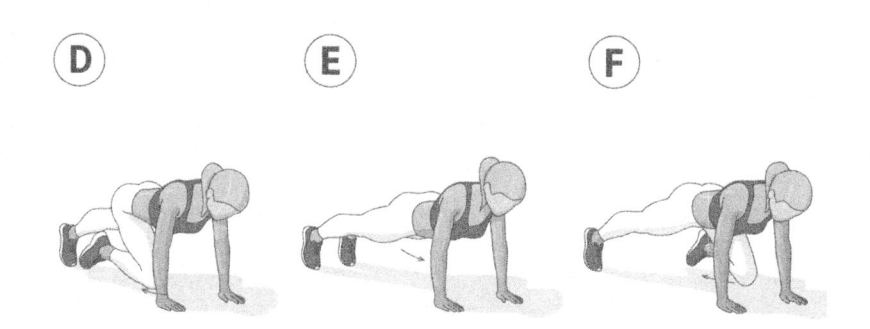

2 - Lunges to Knee Drive: Start standing with feet hip-width apart. Take a step forward with your right foot, bending your knees to lower towards the floor. Then, push your body upward, focusing on the front leg, and bring your left knee towards your chest during the upward push. Alternate sides by taking a step forward with your left foot and bringing your right knee towards your chest during the upward push.

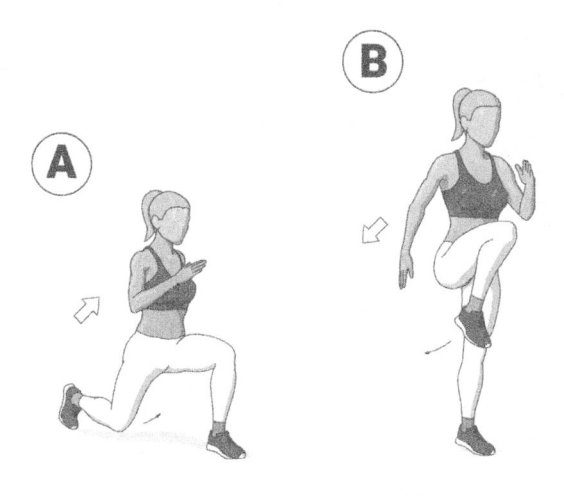

3 - Burpees: Start in a standing position. Perform a push-up, then jump into a squat position, and finally, leap up with arms raised overhead. Repeat the movement throughout the exercise duration.

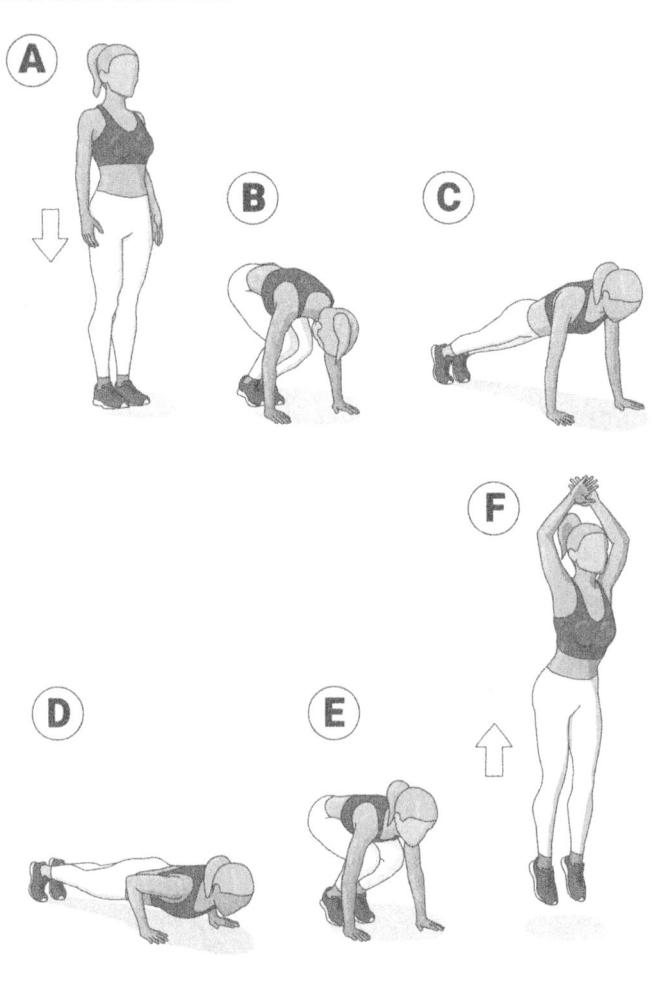

4 - Plank Shoulder Taps: Assume a plank position and alternate tapping your shoulders. This targets your abs, oblique abdominals, and activates the shoulder stabilizers.

→

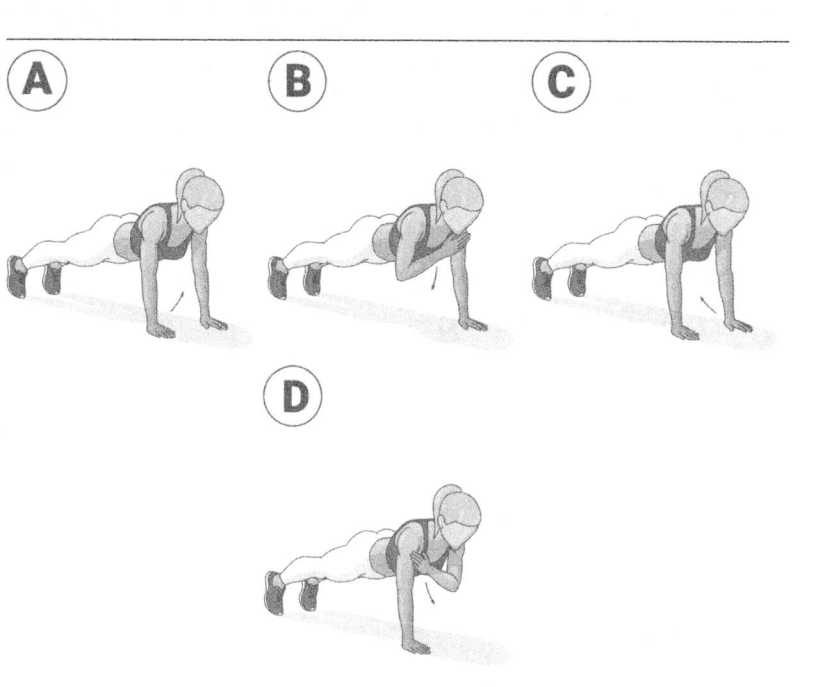

5 - High Knees: Begin in a standing position with arms relaxed at the sides. Take a step forward, raising one knee high towards the chest while simultaneously lifting the opposite arm upward. Quickly alternate legs, maintaining a fast pace and aiming to lift the knees as high as possible. This exercise engages the abs, legs, and improves cardiovascular endurance.

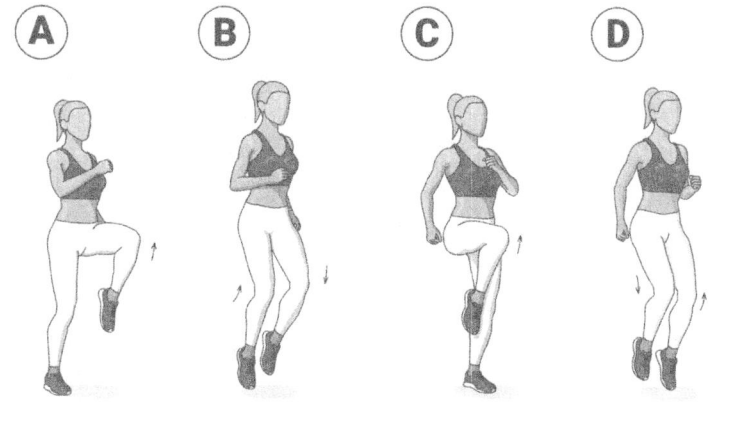

Remember to adjust the intensity of the exercises to your physical abilities and to perform a proper warm-up before starting the workout.

SHEET 4 - GOAL: INTERVAL TRAINING FOR FULL BODY MUSCLE WORK.

45" exercise - 15" active rest = 5 minutes

1 - Jumping Jacks

2 - Traditional Lunges

3 - Plank Walk

4 - Knee to Elbow

5 - Mountain Climbers

EXERCISES AND DESCRIPTIONS:

1 - Jumping Jacks: Begin in a standing position with legs together and arms down at the sides. Then jump, spreading the legs laterally and raising the arms overhead. Return to the starting position and repeat the movement for the entire exercise duration.

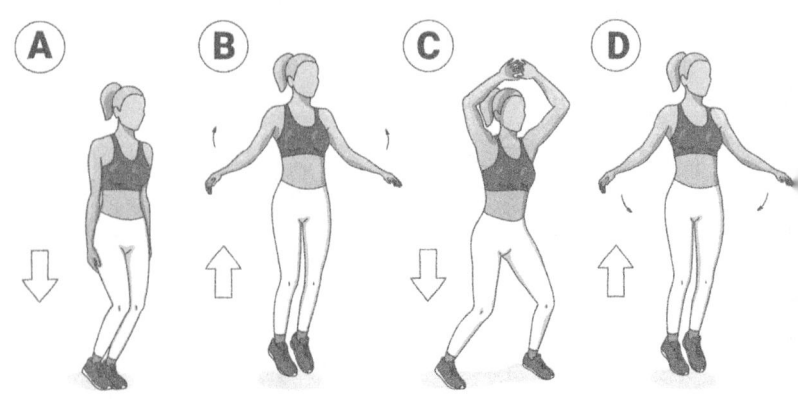

2 - Traditional Lunges: Perform classic lunges, engaging the leg and glute muscles while increasing your heart rate and burning calories.

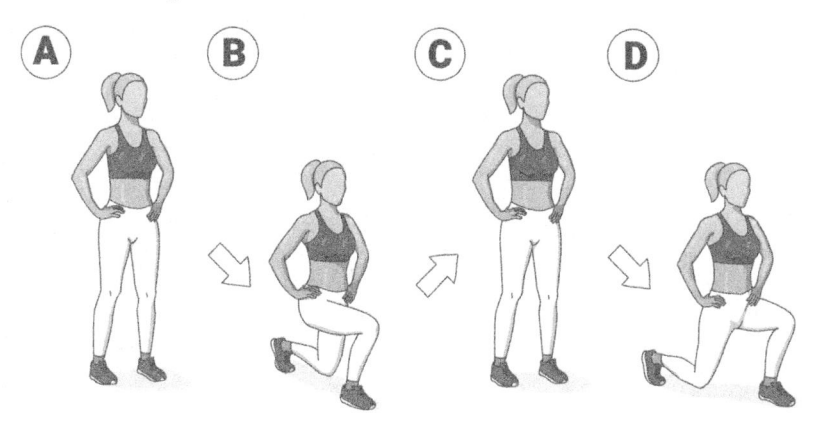

3 - Plank Walk: Engage in a walking movement while in the plank position, involving your core, arms, and legs. This exercise enhances stability and calorie burning.

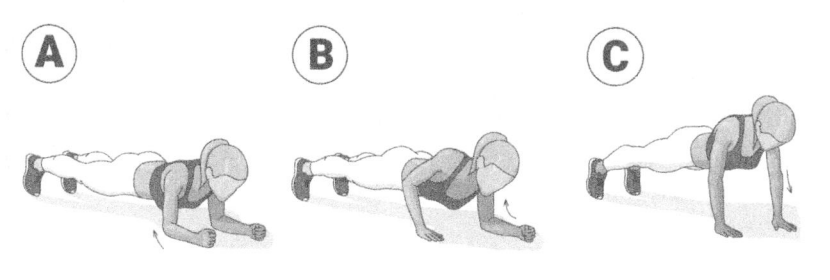

4 - Knee to Elbow: Assume a plank position while bringing your knee close to your elbow. This exercise engages your oblique abdominal muscles and core, promoting fat burning.

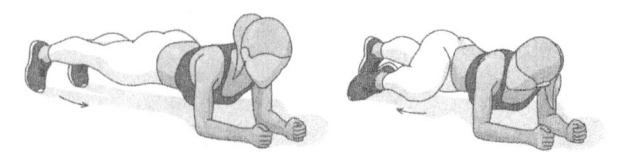

5 - Mountain Climbers: Start in a plank position, then quickly and controlledly bring the knees alternately towards the chest. Keep alternating legs throughout the exercise duration.

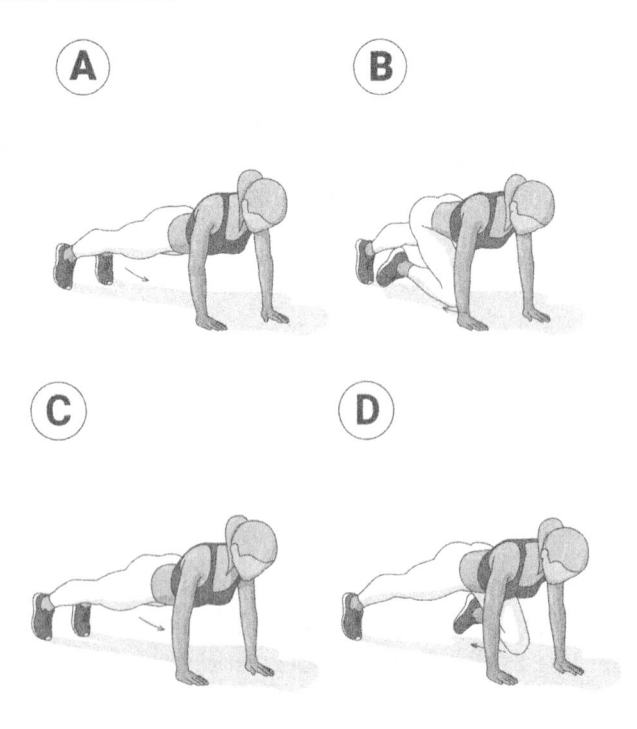

Remember to adjust the intensity of the exercises to your physical abilities and to perform a proper warm-up before starting the workout.

SHEET 5 - GOAL: INTERVAL TRAINING FOR COMPLETE MUSCLE WORKOUT.

45" exercise - 15" active rest = 5 minutes

1 - Burpees

2 - Jump Squats

3 - Plank

4 - Crunches

5 - Plank Walk

EXERCISES AND DESCRIPTIONS:

1 - Burpees: Start in a standing position. Perform a push-up, then jump into a squat position, and finally, leap up with arms raised overhead. Repeat the movement throughout the exercise duration.

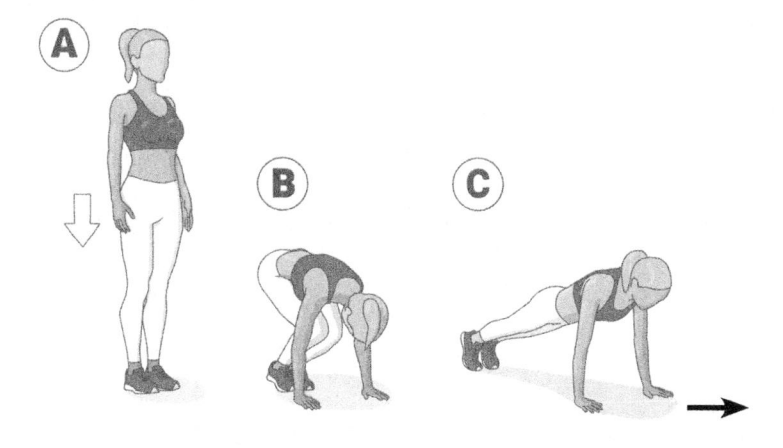

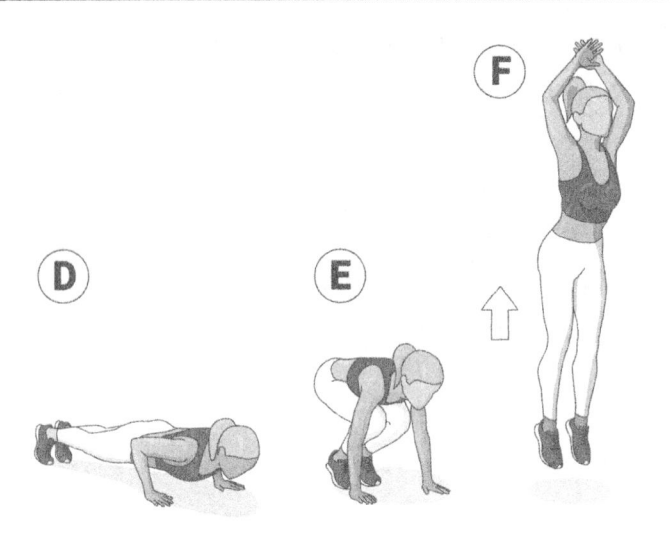

2 - Jump Squats: Perform a squat followed by a high jump. This activates leg, glute, and abdominal muscles, boosting endurance and calorie burn.

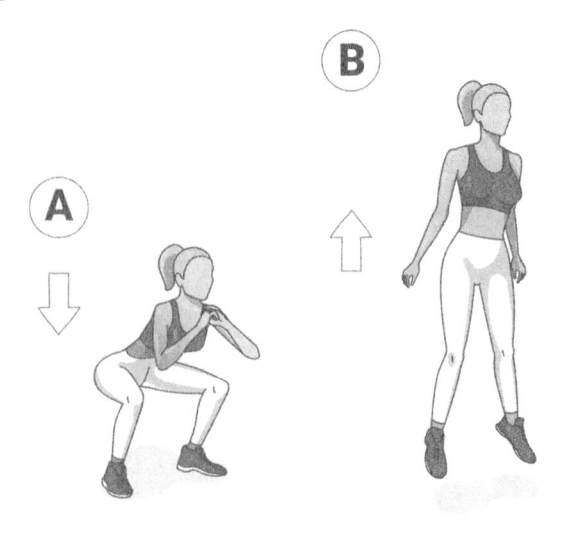

3 - Plank: Assume a static plank position, engaging your abdominal, leg, and arm muscles while stabilizing your core. You can choose between the two options provided.

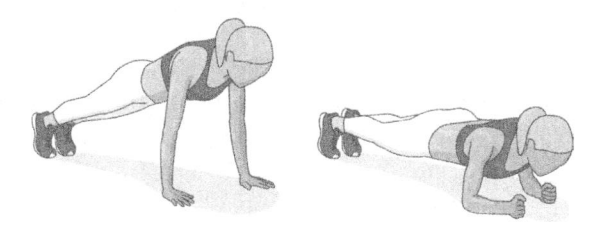

4 - Crunches (Abdominals): You can choose the type of abdominal exercise you prefer, such as crunches, sit-ups, or bicycle crunches. Focus on engaging your abdominal muscles and maintain proper form.

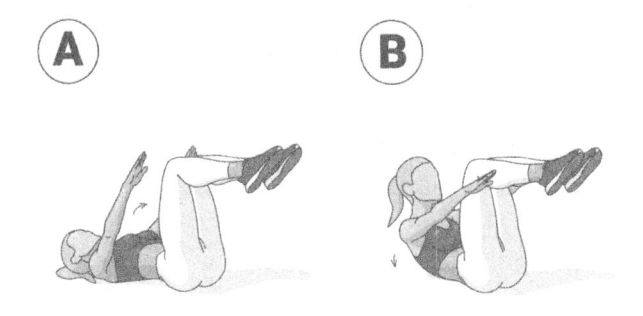

(A) (B)

5 - Plank Walk: Engage in a walking movement while in the plank position, involving your core, arms, and legs. This exercise enhances stability and calorie burning.

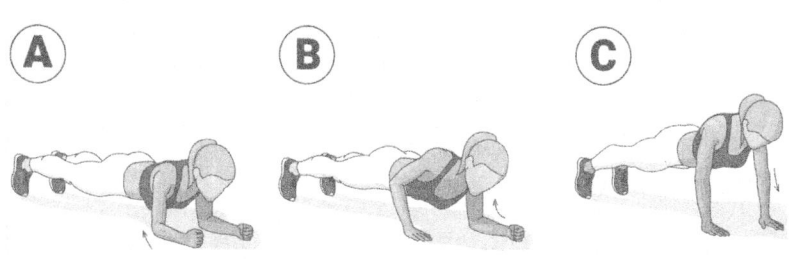

(A) (B) (C)

Remember to adjust the intensity of the exercises to your physical abilities and to perform a proper warm-up before starting the workout.

At the end of this session, I feel exhausted but satisfied for having worked on all muscle groups and achieved an intense cardio activity. Remember to perform each exercise with correct technique and to adapt the intensity based on your abilities.

Session 5: Advanced HIIT Workout to Challenge Your Limits

In session 5, I push myself beyond my limits with an advanced HIIT workout. This session is designed to test my endurance, strength, and agility. Here's how I structure my session:

Description: During this session, I perform a series of high-intensity exercises with short periods of rest. The goal is to work at a sustained pace and put my body under pressure to achieve optimal results.

Timing: Each exercise is performed for 50 seconds, followed by 10 seconds of active recovery. I complete the circuit of exercises in 5 minutes.

Difficulty: This session is suitable for those who already have a good fitness foundation and want to challenge themselves further. The exercises are intense and require a high level of physical and mental commitment. Choose a difficulty level that allows you to work at a sustained pace but is still manageable for you.

Exercise Order: You can follow the order of exercises proposed below or modify it according to your preferences:

SHEET 1 - GOAL: ADVANCED HIIT WORKOUT TO CHALLENGE YOUR LIMITS.

50" exercise - 10" active rest = 5 minutes

1 - Burpees with push-up

2 - Jumping Lunges

3 - Fast-paced mountain climbers

4 - Jump squats with twist

5 - Plank jack with push-up

EXERCISES AND DESCRIPTIONS:

1 - Burpees with push-up: Start standing, perform a push-up on the ground, jump into a squat position, execute a push-up, and then jump up with arms overhead. Repeat the movement for the entire duration of the exercise.

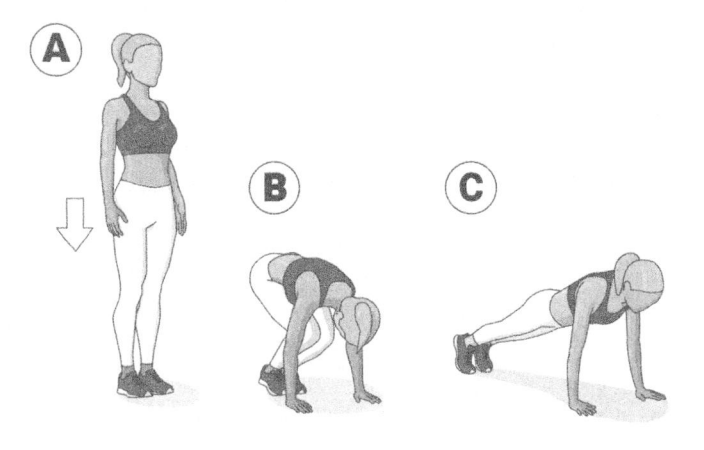

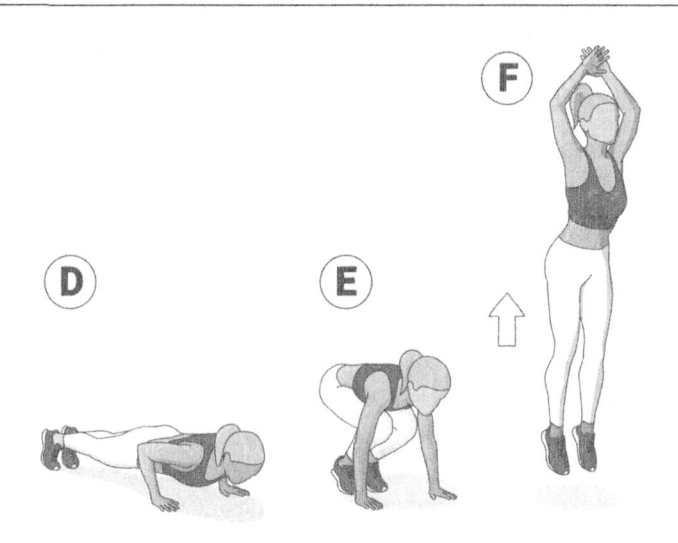

2 - Jumping Lunges: Start in a standing position with one foot forward and the other back in a lunge position. Jump, switching the positions of the legs, so that the foot that was forward is now back, and vice versa. Keep switching legs with a fast and controlled jump.

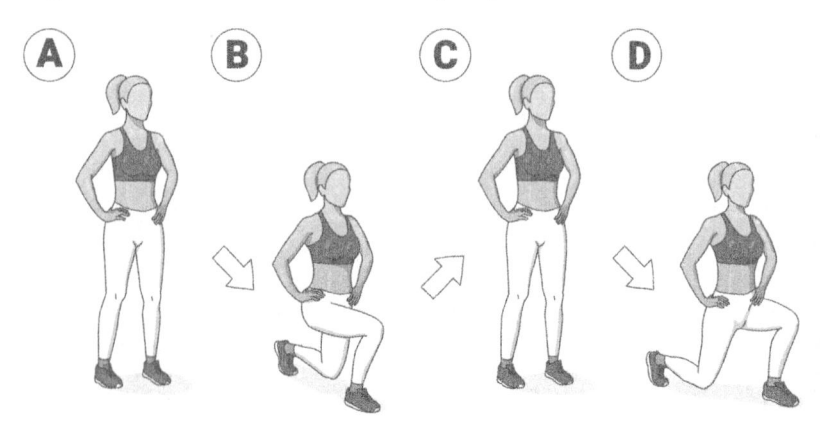

3 - Fast-paced mountain climbers: Get into a plank position, with arms extended and the body in a straight line. Bring your knees toward your chest at a fast pace, maintaining quick and controlled movements. Continue performing mountain climbers for the entire duration of the exercise.

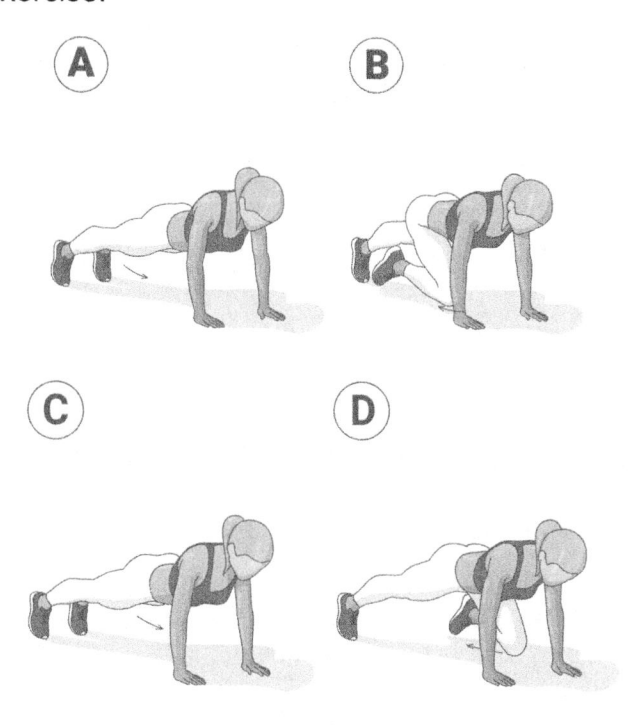

4 - Jump squats with twist: Start standing with your feet slightly wider than shoulder-width apart. Jump up, rotate your body 180 degrees in the air, and land while twisting in the opposite direction. Repeat the movement for the entire duration of the exercise.

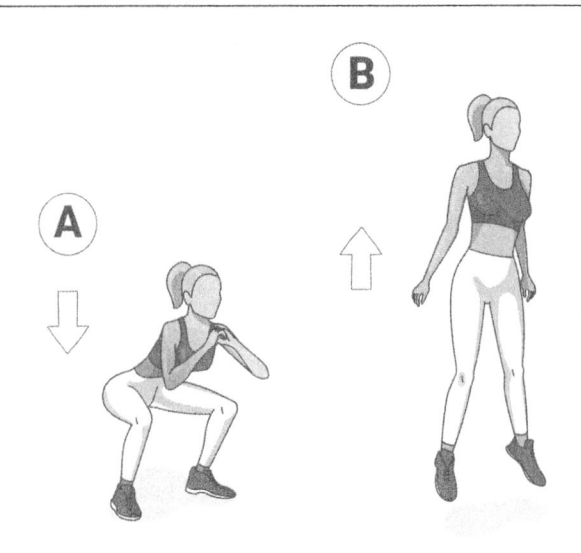

5 - Plank Jack with Push-up: Position yourself in a plank position, with arms extended and the body in a straight line. Jump your feet apart, then perform a push-up. Repeat the movement smoothly for the entire duration of the exercise.

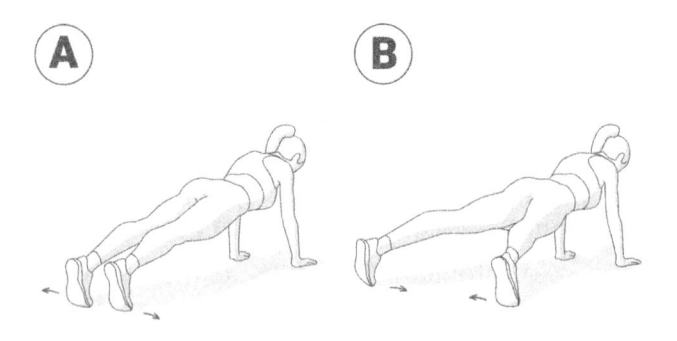

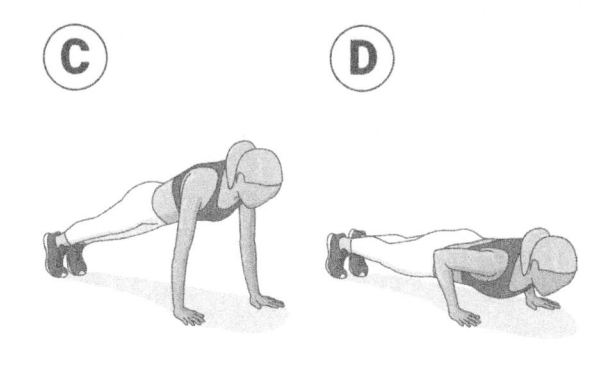

Remember to adjust the intensity of the exercises to your physical abilities and perform a proper warm-up before starting the workout.

SHEET 2 - GOAL: ADVANCED HIIT WORKOUT TO CHALLENGE YOUR LIMITS.

50" exercise - 10" active rest = 5 minutes

1 - Jump Squats

2 - Lunges to Knee Drive

3 - High-Speed Mountain Climbers

4 - Jumping Jacks

5 - Plank Jack with Push-Up

EXERCISES AND DESCRIPTIONS:

1 - Jump Squats: Perform a squat followed by a high jump. This activates leg, glute, and abdominal muscles, boosting endurance and calorie burn.

→

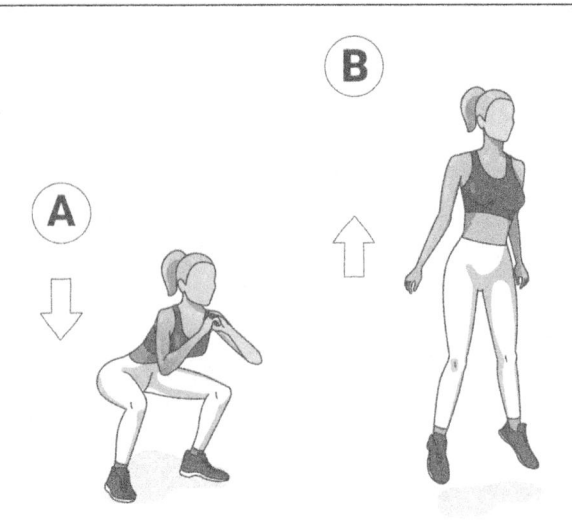

2 - Lunges to Knee Drive: Start standing with feet hip-width apart. Take a step forward with your right foot, bending your knees to lower towards the floor. Then, push your body upward, focusing on the front leg, and bring your left knee towards your chest during the upward push. Alternate sides by taking a step forward with your left foot and bringing your right knee towards your chest during the upward push.

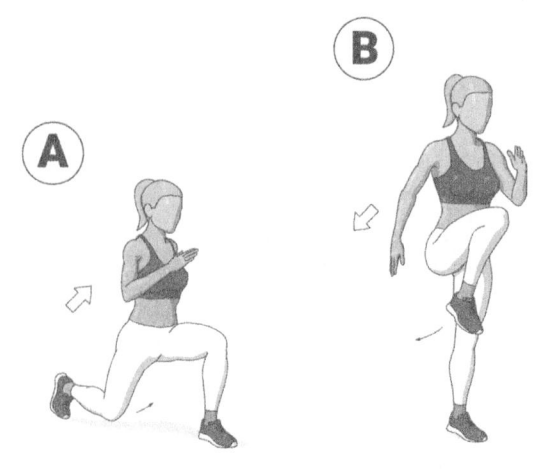

3 - High-Speed Mountain Climbers: Position yourself in a plank position with your arms extended and your body in a straight line. Bring your knees toward your chest quickly, maintaining a rapid and controlled movement. Continue to perform mountain climbers for the entire duration of the exercise.

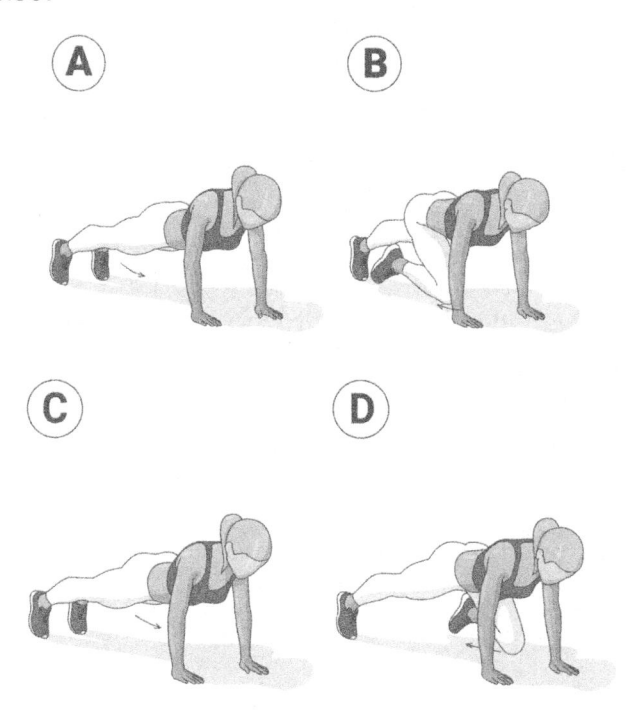

4 - Jumping Jacks: Begin in a standing position with legs together and arms down at the sides. Then jump, spreading the legs laterally and raising the arms overhead. Return to the starting position and repeat the movement for the entire exercise duration.

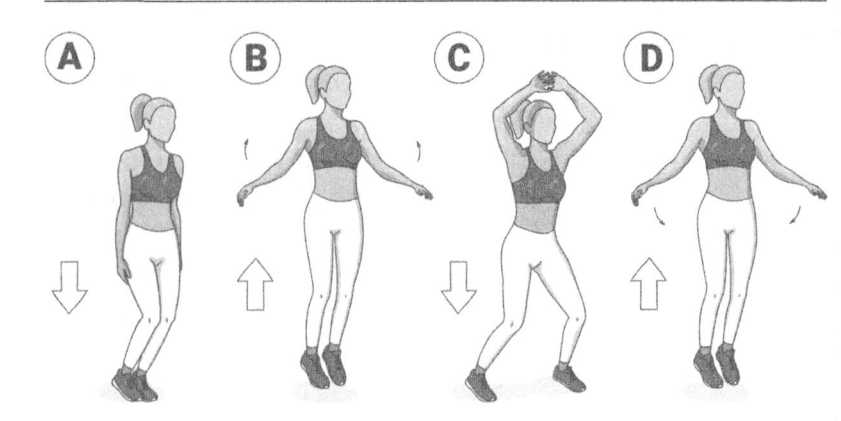

5 - Plank Jack with Push-up: Position yourself in a plank position, with arms extended and the body in a straight line. Jump your feet apart, then perform a push-up. Repeat the movement smoothly for the entire duration of the exercise.

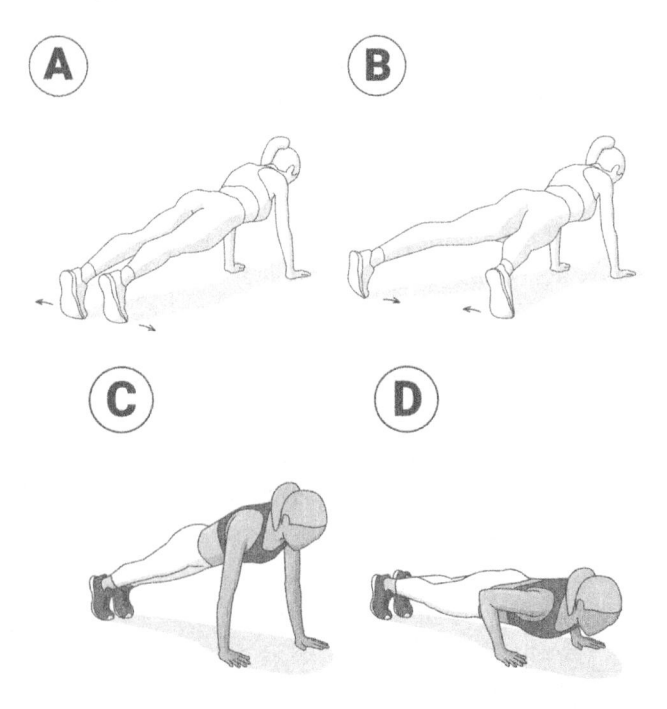

Remember to adjust the intensity of the exercises to your physical capabilities and to perform a proper warm-up before starting the workout.

SHEET 3 - GOAL: ADVANCED HIIT WORKOUT TO CHALLENGE YOUR LIMITS.

50" exercise - 10" active rest = 5 minutes

1 - Burpees with Push-Up

2 - Push-Ups with Mountain Climbers

3 - Jump Squats

4 - Lunges

5 - Plank

EXERCISES AND DESCRIPTIONS:

1 - Burpees with push-up: Start standing, perform a push-up on the ground, jump into a squat position, execute a push-up, and then jump up with arms overhead. Repeat the movement for the entire duration of the exercise.

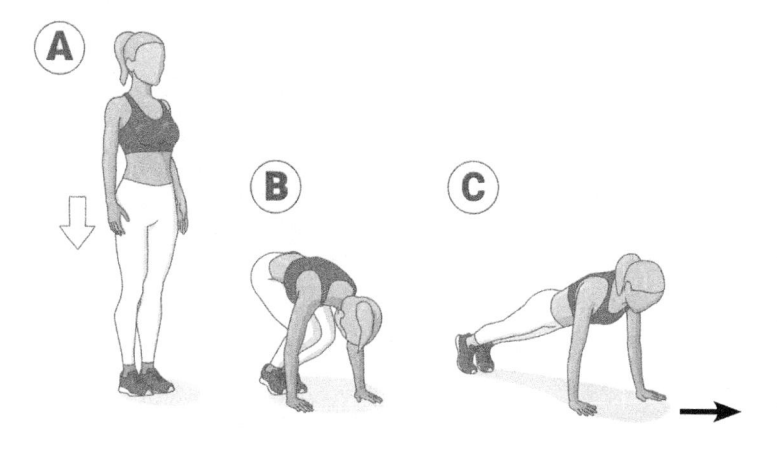

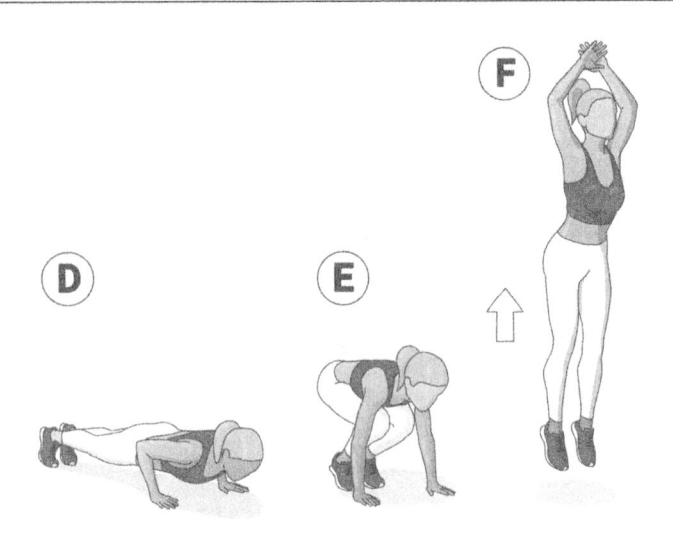

2 - Push-Ups with Mountain Climbers: Do push-ups with mountain climbers for 40 seconds. Perform a push-up on the ground, then when returning to the plank position, alternately bring your right knee and left knee towards your chest, maintaining a fast pace. Continue alternating legs for the entire duration of the exercise.

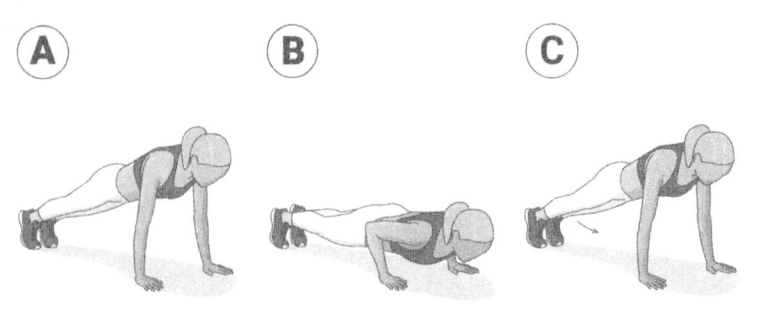

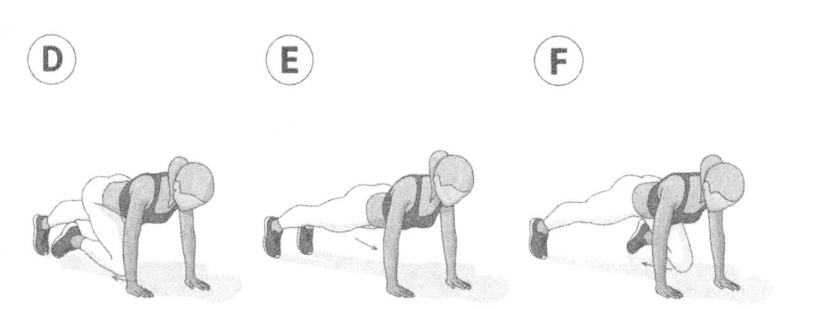

3 - Jump Squats: Perform a squat followed by a high jump. This activates leg, glute, and abdominal muscles, boosting endurance and calorie burn.

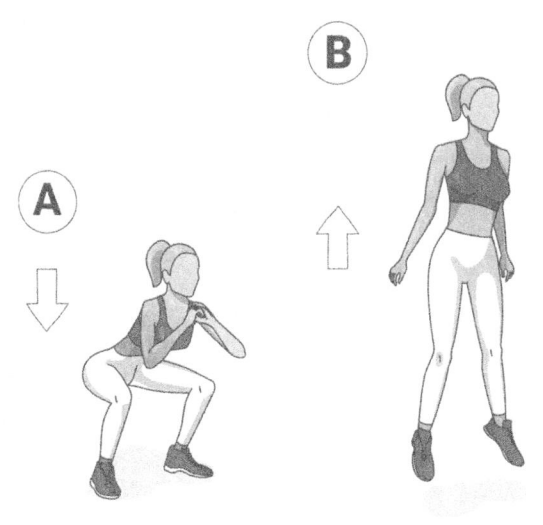

4 - Lunges: Perform classic lunges, engaging the leg and glute muscles while increasing your heart rate and burning calories.

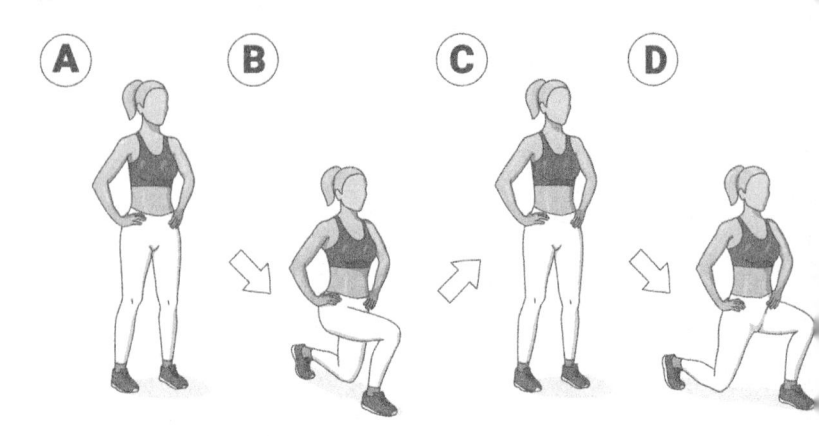

5 - Plank: Assume a static plank position, engaging your abdominal, leg, and arm muscles while stabilizing your core. You can choose between the two options provided.

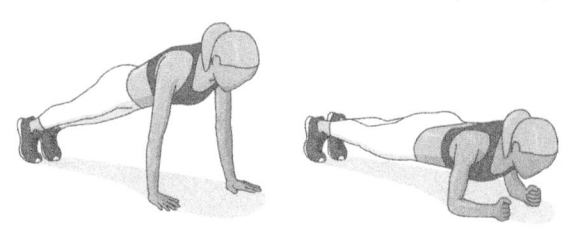

Remember to adjust the intensity of the exercises to your physical abilities and perform a proper warm-up before starting the workout.

SHEET 4 - GOAL: ADVANCED HIIT TRAINING TO CHALLENGE YOUR LIMITS.

50" exercise - 10" active rest = 5 minutes

1 - Jumping Jacks

2 - High-Speed Mountain Climbers

3 - Burpees with Push-Up

4 - Jump Squats

5 - Plank Jack with Push-Up

EXERCISES AND DESCRIPTIONS:

1 - Jumping Jacks: Begin in a standing position with legs together and arms down at the sides. Then jump, spreading the legs laterally and raising the arms overhead. Return to the starting position and repeat the movement for the entire exercise duration.

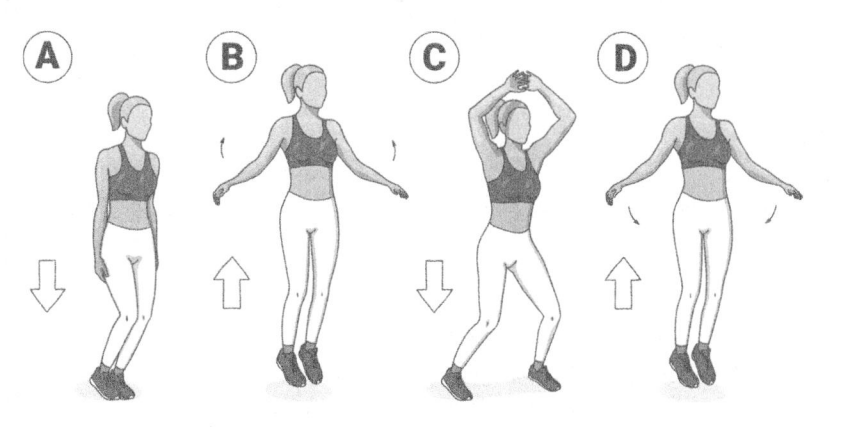

2 - High-Speed Mountain Climbers: Position yourself in a plank position with your arms extended and your body in a straight line. Bring your knees toward your chest quickly, maintaining a rapid and controlled movement. Continue to perform mountain climbers for the entire duration of the exercise.

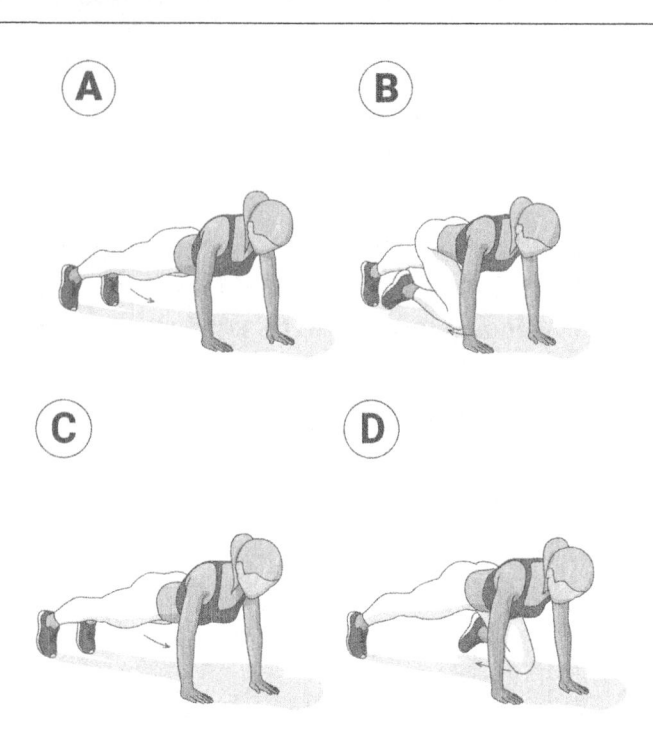

3 - Burpees with push-up: Start standing, perform a push-up on the ground, jump into a squat position, execute a push-up, and then jump up with arms overhead. Repeat the movement for the entire duration of the exercise.

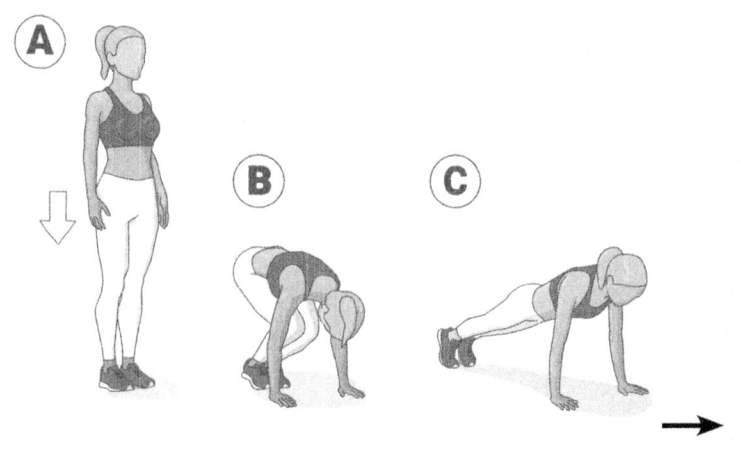

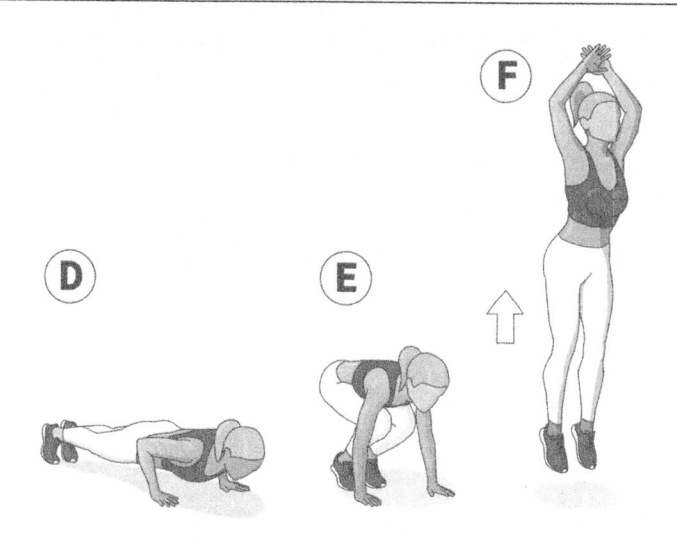

4 - Jump Squats: Perform a squat followed by a high jump. This activates leg, glute, and abdominal muscles, boosting endurance and calorie burn.

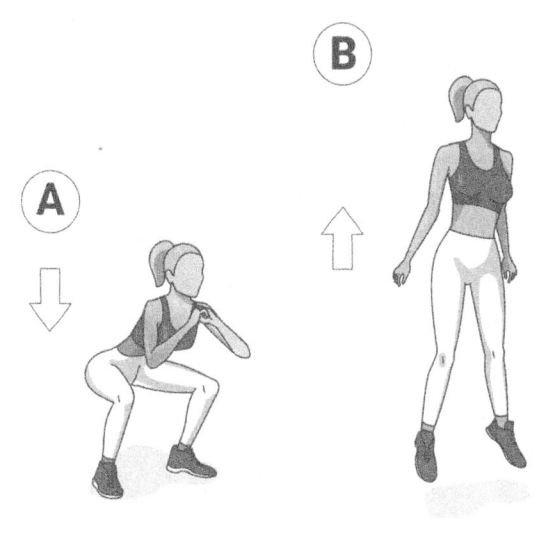

5 - Plank Jack with Push-up: Position yourself in a plank position, with arms extended and the body in a straight line. Jump your feet apart, then perform a push-up. Repeat the movement smoothly for the entire duration of the exercise.

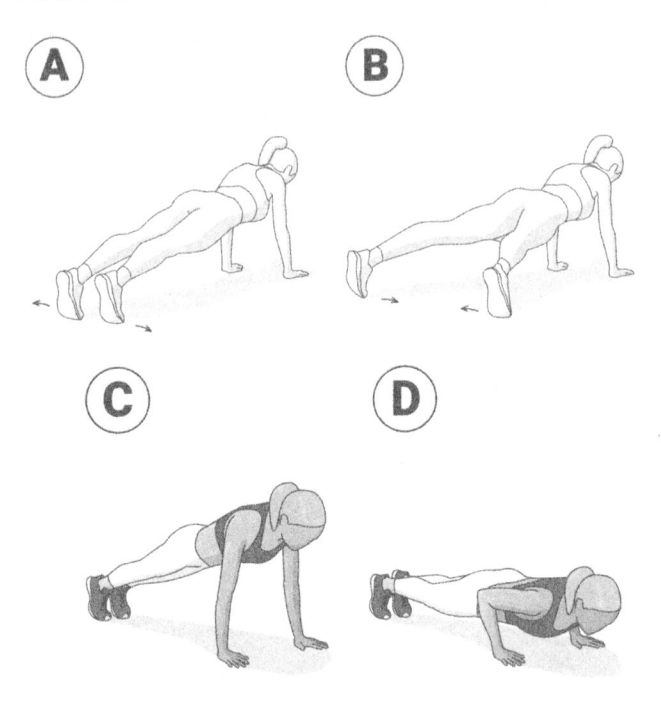

Remember to adjust the intensity of the exercises according to your physical abilities and to perform a proper warm-up before starting the workout.

SHEET 5 - GOAL: ADVANCED HIIT WORKOUT TO CHALLENGE YOUR LIMITS.

50" exercise - 10" active rest = 5 minutes

1 - Lunges to Knee Drive

2 - Plank Jack with Push-Up

3 - Jump Squats

4 - High-Speed Mountain Climbers

5 - Burpees with Push-Up

EXERCISES AND DESCRIPTIONS:

1 - Lunges to Knee Drive: Start standing with feet hip-width apart. Take a step forward with your right foot, bending your knees to lower towards the floor. Then, push your body upward, focusing on the front leg, and bring your left knee towards your chest during the upward push. Alternate sides by taking a step forward with your left foot and bringing your right knee towards your chest during the upward push.

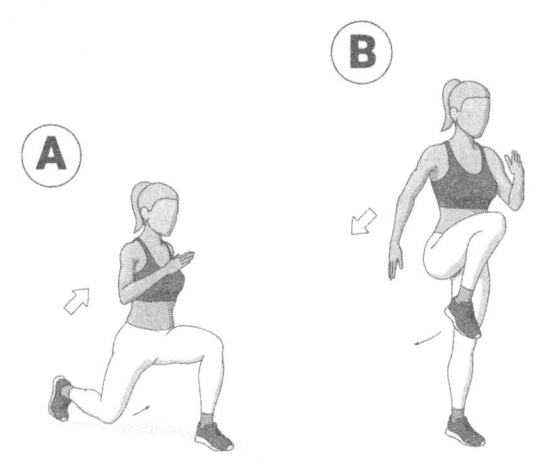

2 - Plank Jack with Push-up: Position yourself in a plank position, with arms extended and the body in a straight line. Jump your feet apart, then perform a push-up. Repeat the movement smoothly for the entire duration of the exercise.

→

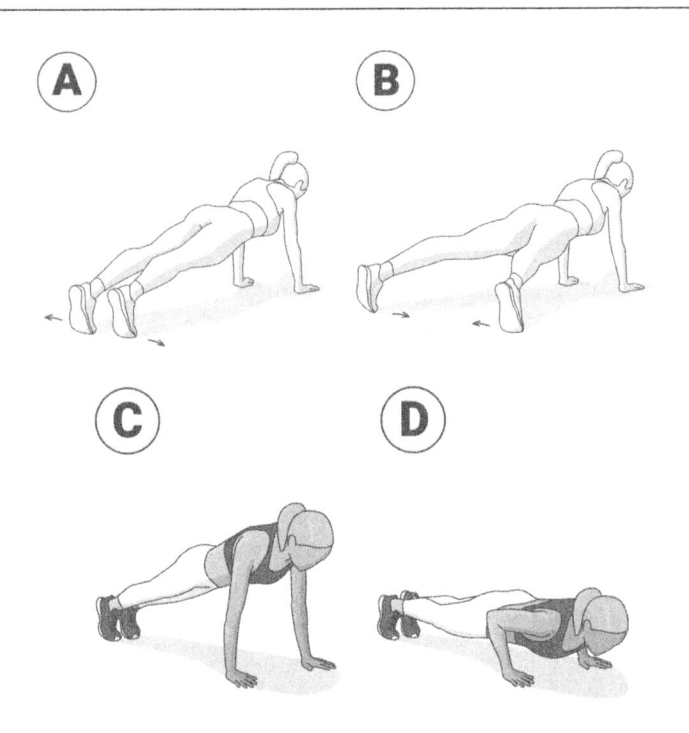

3 - Jump Squats: Perform a squat followed by a high jump. This activates leg, glute, and abdominal muscles, boosting endurance and calorie burn.

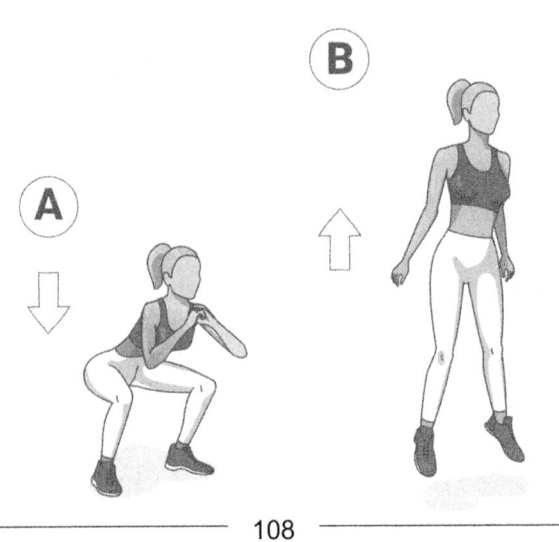

4 - High-Speed Mountain Climbers: Position yourself in a plank position with your arms extended and your body in a straight line. Bring your knees toward your chest quickly, maintaining a rapid and controlled movement. Continue to perform mountain climbers for the entire duration of the exercise.

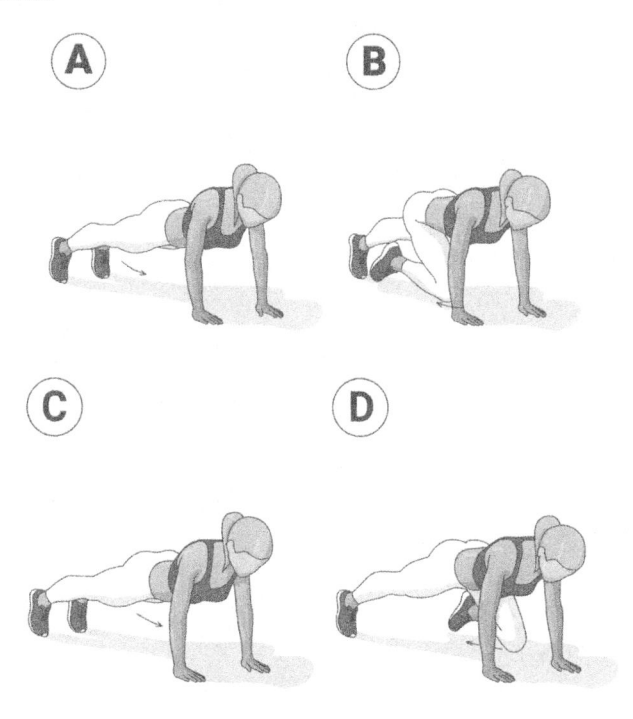

(A) (B)

(C) (D)

5 - Burpees with push-up: Start standing, perform a push-up on the ground, jump into a squat position, execute a push-up, and then jump up with arms overhead. Repeat the movement for the entire duration of the exercise.

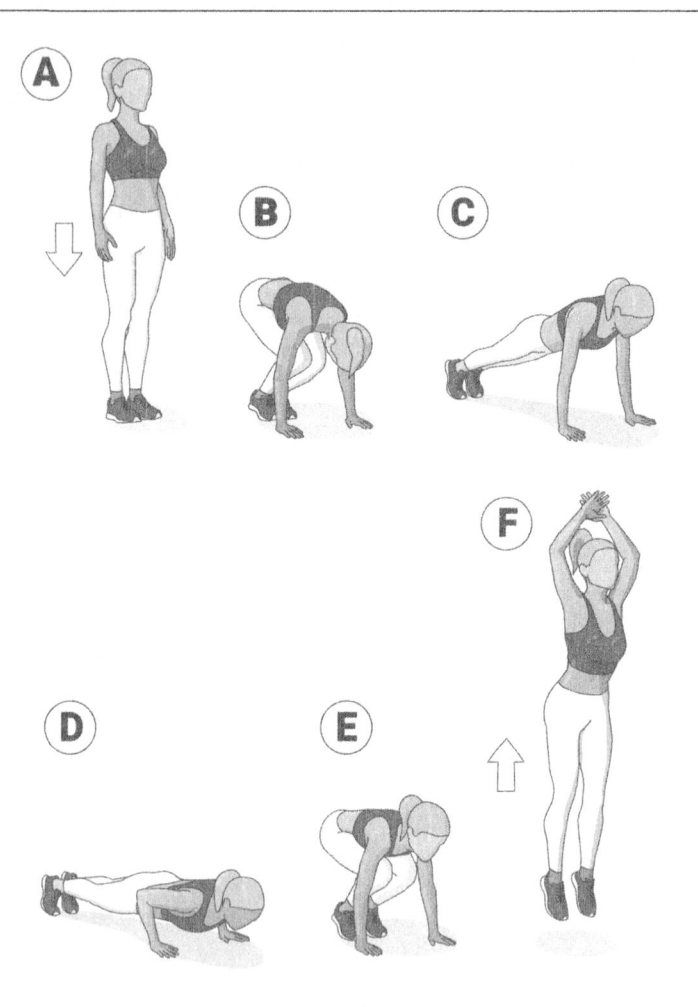

Remember to adjust the intensity of the exercises according to your physical abilities and to perform a proper warm-up before starting the workout.

This advanced session of HIIT training is a true test of endurance and strength. Make sure to perform each exercise with proper technique and adjust the intensity according to your capabilities. Challenge yourself and push to the maximum to achieve extraordinary results.

CHAPTER 4: TRACKING YOUR PROGRESS

In Chapter 4 of my HIIT training body toning journey, I emphasize the importance of monitoring progress. **Keeping tabs on my achievements plays a crucial role in assessing improvements, staying motivated, and adapting my workout plan as needed.**

Here's how I tackle the task of progress tracking.

In this chapter, I explore various methods for recording my results and monitoring my performance over time. I employ tools like workout journals, tracking apps, body measurements, and performance tests to obtain a comprehensive view of my progress.

I make a commitment to regularly monitor my workouts and progress. I diligently document the specifics of each workout session, including factors like intensity, duration, and the exercises performed. Moreover, I keep a keen eye on improvements such as enhanced endurance, reduced recovery times, and increased strength.

For effective results tracking, I utilize either a workout journal or a dedicated app. These aids enable me to maintain an organized record of past workouts, track my progress over time, and spot trends or areas where further improvements are possible.

In addition to tracking performance, I also measure changes in my physique. I employ tools such as weight measurements, body circumference assessments, and body composition evaluations to gain a more precise understanding of my progress in terms of toning and weight management.

At regular intervals, I carry out performance tests aimed at assessing my current fitness level and overall progress. These tests may include timed runs, repetitions of specific exercises, or the time taken to complete a workout circuit. These evaluations help me gauge my fitness level at any given moment and set new performance goals accordingly.

Progress tracking offers me a clear and insightful overview of my HIIT training body toning journey. This chapter serves as a valuable tool for recognizing improvements, sustaining motivation, and pinpointing areas in need of refinement.

CHAPTER 5: NUTRITION AND SUPPLEMENTATION

In Chapter 5, I delve into the vital aspects of nutrition and supplementation to fuel my body toning journey through HIIT training. Understanding that proper nutrition plays a pivotal role in achieving the best results and unlocking my full potential is key.

Here's how I tackle the realms of nutrition and supplementation.

Within this chapter, I take a deep dive into the core principles of crafting a well-rounded diet tailored to the demands of HIIT training. I also share practical wisdom on creating a balanced meal plan while underscoring the significance of supplements, encompassing vitamins, minerals, and specialized enhancements to elevate my performance and facilitate muscle recovery.

Balanced Nutrition: I comprehend the significance of maintaining a balanced diet enriched with a diverse array of nourishing foods. My diet ensures an ample intake of protein to stimulate muscle growth, complex carbohydrates to fuel my workouts, and healthy fats for optimal bodily functions. Furthermore, I'm diligent about nourishing my body with vitamins, minerals, and antioxidants obtained from fruits, vegetables, and whole foods.

Hydration: Hydration proves paramount during my HIIT workouts. I make a conscientious effort to remain well-hydrated by consuming an adequate volume of water before, during, and after my exercise sessions, replenishing fluids lost through perspiration. While water remains my primary choice, I'm open to incorporating electrolyte-infused beverages when engaging in high-intensity physical activities.

Strategic Supplementation: Under certain circumstances, I may choose to complement my dietary intake with specific supplements designed to boost performance and expedite muscle recovery. Prior to incorporating any supplements, I conduct thorough research and seek guidance from healthcare professionals to ensure safety and efficacy. Common supplements in my regimen may include protein powders, branched-chain amino acids (BCAAs), or omega-3 supplements.

Mindful Eating: I maintain mindfulness around my dietary habits and make deliberate selections that align with my objectives of body toning. My dietary choices steer clear of ultra-processed, sugary, and saturated fat-laden foods, which encompass packaged snacks, sugary beverages, energy drinks, confectionery treats, sugary cereals, powdered drinks, and canned or jarred ready-made meals. I'm attentive to portion control and endeavor to maintain a balanced and moderate approach to eating throughout the day without overindulging.

Nutrition and supplementation form an integral part of my HIIT training regimen, offering invaluable support in my pursuit of body toning goals. By adhering to a well-structured meal plan, staying adequately hydrated, and making informed supplement choices, I ensure my body receives the essential nutrients required for peak performance and enduring results.

Typically, I adhere to a consistent and well-balanced meal schedule that satisfies my daily energy and nutritional needs. Adhering to dietary guidelines, I consume three principal meals (breakfast, lunch, and dinner) and two intermediary snacks (mid-morning and mid-afternoon) positioned between primary meals.

For me, the core of effective nutrition lies in selecting nutrient-rich foods for all meals and snacks, while being vigilant about steering clear of highly processed, sugary, and saturated fat-laden options. Moreover, I pay heed to my body's cues, respecting signals of hunger and satiety to maintain a harmonious dietary equilibrium.

CHAPTER 6: RECOVERY AND OVERALL WELL-BEING

In Chapter 6 of my journey towards toning my body with HIIT training, I place my focus on recovery and enhancing my overall well-being. **I comprehend the pivotal role that proper rest and well-being practices play in achieving the best possible results and maintaining a harmonious balance in my life.**

Here's how I approach the realms of recovery and nurturing my overall well-being.

Description: Within this chapter, I delve into the significance of post-HIIT workout recovery and share practical strategies aimed at fostering muscle recuperation, relaxation, and a holistic sense of well-being. Additionally, I delve into self-care practices such as stretching, massage, and meditation, all of which contribute to facilitating recovery and diminishing stress.

Active and Passive Rest: I'm well aware of the value of both active and passive forms of rest for my body. Beyond the passive recuperation linked to getting sufficient nightly sleep, I make it a point to incorporate active rest into my training regimen. This might involve active rest days, which encompass activities like yoga or gentle strolls—approaches that encourage recovery without placing undue strain on my muscles.

Muscle Relaxation: Following each HIIT workout session, I allocate time to focus on muscle relaxation. I employ a variety of dynamic and static stretching techniques designed to enhance flexibility and alleviate the accumulated muscle tension resulting from training. This practice serves to preempt potential injuries while promoting the recovery of my muscles.

Self-Care and Active Recovery: I'm diligent in caring for my body by engaging in self-care practices such as self-massage using foam rollers or massage balls. These techniques are instrumental in releasing muscle tension and stimulating blood circulation, thereby expediting healing and promoting optimal recovery.

Stress Management: I place due emphasis on managing stress within my life. Given that HIIT training can exert substantial demands on the body, I'm committed to weaving stress management practices into my daily routine. This includes activities like meditation, deep breathing exercises, or other relaxation methods that contribute to preserving mental and emotional equilibrium, thus elevating my overall sense of well-being.

Body Awareness: I've cultivated a heightened sense of body awareness by diligently heeding my body's cues and responding with prudence. I comprehend the importance of respecting my body's limitations and tailoring both my training and recovery strategies to suit its specific needs. Such awareness enables me to stave off injuries while maintaining an optimum state of overall well-being.

The chapter dedicated to recovery and overall well-being serves as a poignant reminder of the significance of self-care not solely during the training process but also during periods of rest. By striking a balance through adequate rest, muscle relaxation, active recuperation, and stress management, I'm able to maximize the benefits of HIIT training while nurturing a profound sense of holistic well-being that transcends the realm of physical fitness alone.

CHAPTER 7: SUSTAINING LONG-TERM RESULTS

In Chapter 7 of my body sculpting journey with HIIT training, I focus on the art of keeping my achievements intact over the long haul. **I recognize that genuine success doesn't stop at reaching a specific goal; it's about preserving those accomplishments through time.**

Here's how I make sure I maintain long-term results:

Consistency and Dedication: I understand that the golden rule for preserving results is to be **consistent in training**. I pledge to stick to my HIIT workout program faithfully, maintaining my commitment and resolve even after hitting my initial goals. Consistency is the linchpin for preserving and enhancing my fitness over time.

Adaptations and Progressions: I grasp that as time goes on, the body adapts to the training it's subjected to. Therefore, I make it a point to continuously introduce fresh challenges and progressions into my HIIT workout regimen. This might involve amping up the intensity of exercises, mixing up repetition patterns, or incorporating new exercises that activate different muscle groups. Keeping my program dynamic and stimulating is my secret to staying motivated and consistently witnessing results.

Balance and Diversity: To prevent fatigue and potential plateaus in my progress, I ensure that my HIIT training is balanced with other forms of physical activity. I also weave active recovery periods into my routine. I actively explore various activities such as yoga, swimming, or cycling to maintain diversity and stimulate my body in different ways.

Balanced Nutrition: I'm acutely aware of how crucial a balanced and nutritious diet is in supporting the gains I've made through HIIT training. I commit to following a healthy eating plan brimming with essential nutrients that fuel my workouts and promote muscle recovery. My aim is to uphold a harmonious blend of carbohydrates, proteins, and healthy fats while embracing a rich variety of fruits, vegetables, and whole foods.

Positive Mindset and Motivation: The power of the mind in sustaining results is something I don't underestimate. I vow to nurture a positive mindset, keep my motivation high, and set my sights on long-term objectives. Visualization techniques, affirmative self-talk, and the support of like-minded individuals all play a role in keeping me motivated on my body sculpting journey.

The chapter on maintaining long-term results serves as a reminder that the real test is about unwavering consistency and an unyielding pursuit of improvement. Through commitment, diversity, wholesome nutrition, and a positive mindset, I can safeguard the results achieved through HIIT training over time and bask in the enduring health and wellness benefits.

CONCLUSION

Throughout this journey of body toning with HIIT training, I've come to realize that dedicating just 5 minutes a day can yield remarkable results. High-Intensity Interval Training has served as my invaluable tool for shedding excess fat, sculpting lean muscles, and achieving a finely tuned level of physical fitness.

By delving into the fundamental principles of HIIT, understanding the structure of workout sessions, and paying close attention to my nutrition and rest, I've achieved impressive outcomes. I've witnessed noticeable enhancements in my endurance, strength, and overall body composition.

The practice of tracking my progress has played a pivotal role in helping me monitor results and tailor my training regimen accordingly. I've cultivated consistency, continuously embraced fresh challenges, and struck a harmonious balance between rigorous training and holistic well-being.

But this adventure doesn't conclude here. Sustaining long-term results necessitates unwavering commitment and persistent dedication. I fully grasp that the journey towards a toned and healthy physique is an enduring one, and I stand prepared to continually push my boundaries and exceed my own expectations.

Armed with a positive mindset, unshakable motivation, and a crystal-clear awareness of my objectives, I'm confident in my ability to attain and preserve peak physical fitness. HIIT training has seamlessly woven itself into the fabric of my life, delivering not only visible results but also a heightened sense of self-assurance and an overall boost in well-being.

I'm immensely grateful for embarking on this transformative journey, and I extend an encouraging invitation to anyone seeking to experience the benefits of HIIT training, which can sculpt your body in just 5 minutes a day. Regardless of your starting point, with steadfast commitment and unyielding perseverance, you can reach your goals and revel in the myriad advantages that HIIT training has to offer.

AUTHOR INFORMATION

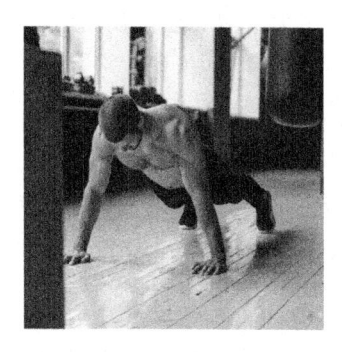

Greetings, everyone! I'm **Lenry Lombardo** (my stage name), an ardent athlete who derives immense joy from physical training.

I want to share my extensive experiences in the realm of sports training and all the valuable insights I've gathered along my journey.

Sports constitute an indispensable facet of my life, an endeavor that not only fuels my spirit but also compels me to perpetually surpass my own boundaries.

I firmly believe that training transcends being merely a physical pursuit; it serves as an opportunity to unearth our inner reservoirs of strength, surmount our preconceived limitations, and forge a profound connection with ourselves.

My aim is to convey the exhilaration I've experienced throughout this journey, chronicling the tribulations, triumphs, and invaluable lessons that have enriched my path. I aspire for my words to kindle a fire within you, inspiring you to conquer your personal hurdles and scale new pinnacles in your own training expedition.

Irrespective of your current proficiency level or aspirations, my hope is that my words shall serve as both a compass and a reliable companion along your odyssey. I aspire to be your confidant, your fellow sojourner, poised to bolster your spirit when challenges seem insurmountable and to jubilate alongside you with each modest victory.

Are you prepared to embark on this odyssey with me? Extend your virtual hand, and let us journey together into the realm of discovery, personal evolution, and triumph through athletic training. Together, we can surmount the most formidable obstacles, stretch our capabilities to the brink, and achieve feats that once seemed beyond reach.

I'm elated to share my adventures with you and witness the remarkable feats we can achieve in unison! Brace yourselves to push your limits, endeavor to discover your untapped potential, and prepare for an exhilarating adventure.

Are we poised for this thrilling expedition? I'm eagerly anticipating the commencement of this journey together!

Printed in Great Britain
by Amazon